To Bukella —
My Thanks for the
Unique Blend of Emotion
Your Style [?]

D1300369

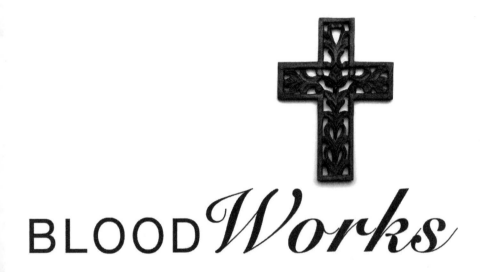

BLOOD*Works*

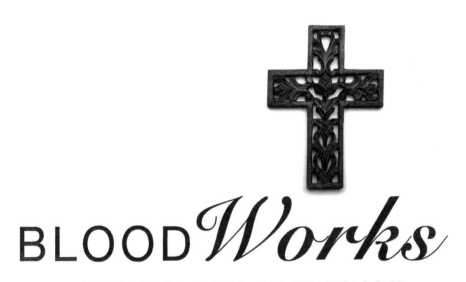

BLOOD *Works*

THE INSIGHTS OF A PASTOR AND HEMATOLOGIST
INTO THE WONDER AND SPIRITUAL POWER OF BLOOD

BISHOP HORACE E. SMITH, M.D.
FOREWORD BY DR. LEIGHTON FORD

Formatting and jacket design by Anne McLaughlin, Blue Lake Design, Dickinson, Texas
Published in the United States by Baxter Press.

ISBN: 978-1-888237-41-2

This book is dedicated to those who gave me life, nurtured my faith, and instilled in me a drive for knowledge and excellence. To my parents, Albert and Shirley Smith, whose DNA I and my siblings proudly carry. To my grandmother, Alberta Pryor, who instilled in me a fervent love for Christ, the church, and the hymns of the faith. To my first pastor, Bishop John S. Holly, who convinced me that faith and science were intimately connected and supported my nascent dreams to become a practitioner of both. All have gone to be with the Lord, but each has entrusted to me a rich heritage that I cherish daily.

I also dedicate this book to my Lord and Savior Jesus Christ, whose precious blood continually and eternally gives life to us all.

Contents

Acknowledgements

This book is the product of the heart and skills of many different people. I want to thank . . .

The Apostolic Faith Church family, where I have been a member for 50 years and who I have been blessed to pastor for thirty years. My faith that anything is possible has been formed and nurtured in your rich soil. You have supported all my endeavors in faith and science. I deeply value our relationship.

My pastor and mentor, Bishop Arthur M. Brazier, whose cosmopolitan life of faith, service, and excellence I continue to try to emulate.

Dr. Samuel Chand, life consultant and dream releaser, who listened to my vision for this book over ten years ago and kept reminding me that it must be completed and shared.

Pat Springle of Baxter Press, who listened carefully to my heart and helped formulate and direct this project to its conclusion. Your expertise and guidance was indispensable.

My wonderful and gifted daughters, Lauren Elrod, Rachel Horton, and Emily Green—and their spouses, my three sons—who have gracefully shared their father with so many others.

Susan Davenport Smith, my wife, companion, closest friend, and courageous critic, who loves me deeply, listens to my heart, and enriches every aspect of my life.

My colleagues in ministry and hematology, who keep me inspired and motivated.

Foreword

My brother-in-law Billy Graham has said he wishes he could preach one more time. If he did, his message would come from Paul's words: "God forbid that I should boast, save in the cross of our Lord Jesus Christ." In this fine book, Horace Smith helps us see why the cross is so central, because it was there that the cleansing blood of Jesus was shed to set us free.

There is a thread, writes poet William Stafford, which runs through things that change, but the thread itself doesn't change. That thread, believes Horace Smith, is blood—blood which is the very stuff of life itself.

The book we call the Bible tells us that God has spoken to us through nature—"the heavens declare the glory of God," through our human nature—"we are fearfully and wonderfully made" writes the Psalmist, and through the Story which runs throughout the Bible, the story that ties together creation and the new creation, and which centers in the coming of God's own Son in our own human likeness—in a body of flesh *and blood.*

And one of the most important things God tells us is that life— the life of the flesh and the soul—is in the blood.

Dr. Horace Smith is uniquely qualified to write of the marvelous power of blood, being both a physician of the body, as a hematologist, and a curate of the soul, as a pastor and bishop of his church. I have known Horace Smith as an intelligent and valuable member of the board of World Vision, on which we both serve, and as a warm, loving, and fun-loving human being. What I did not realize fully until I began to read this book is what a gifted teacher he is of God's Word. His ability to articulate God's truth has been evident from the clarity of the Bible-based devotions he has provided at our board meetings, along with a physician's ability to diagnose our ills. His medical students at Northwestern University have certainly recognized his skill as a teacher. Now, as we read this book, we can see how his congregation in Chicago has benefited from a similar gift of teaching from the pulpit where he has preached for many years.

This book is fascinating to me because of the reality which Bishop Smith attaches to both body and spirit, not denying either. It is full of intriguing facts of how our bodies work. I was amazed to learn that there are forty million miles of channels that carry blood through our bodies! And that there are fifty billion sentries and soldiers in our bodies—we call them white cells—on guard against disease.

Equally wonderful, Dr. Smith reminds us is that these white cells are a powerful metaphor of how God protects us, and that through the blood God's Son shed on the cross, God directs all his love and compassion toward us.

Two stories about the power of blood, from two ends of our human social spectrum, came to me as I read this book. One is a recording made (by accident) by a radio station in England of an old homeless man near a train station in London singing, over and over and over, "Never failed me yet, never failed me yet, Jesus' blood never failed me yet." That song, recorded, played and replayed, became a national hit and brought the message of Jesus' redeeming love to millions who otherwise never would have given it a thought.

The other story of the power of blood is the testimony of the president of Fuller Seminary, Richard Mouw, who recalls that during his doctoral studies his mind had outgrown his heart. Then one day—also in Horace Smith's Chicago—he turned on his radio and

heard the Moody Chorale sing a hymn he had often heard as a boy
growing up in his New Jersey church: "Nothing but the Blood of
Jesus." His heart was renewed as he realized that nothing his mind
could fathom could match the miraculous life-giving power of Jesus'
blood.

I believe—and pray—that this book will both inform your mind
and inspire your heart. And I pray that, in the words of Charles Wesley's great hymn, you will exclaim, "And can it be, that I should gain,
an interest in my Savior's blood."

Leighton Ford, President
Leighton Ford Ministries
Charlotte, North Carolina

Preface

When physicians examine patients, whether it's for a routine physical or a life-threatening disease, perhaps the most common diagnostic tool is a blood test. The doctor typically turns to the nurse or physician's assistant and says, "Get me the following blood work on this patient." Then the doctor lists the specific tests he wants to conduct. Testing the person's blood uncovers previously hidden truths about the health or pathology of every part of the person's physiology. Blood work can reveal the presence of disease or other abnormalities affecting an organ or system. These tests are indispensable to the doctor's diagnosis and treatment plan for the individual.

In the spiritual world, God invites us to test our faith and his nature to uncover previously hidden truths. Paul instructs us, "Examine yourselves to see whether you are in the faith; test yourselves" (2 Corinthians 13:5). And David invites us, "Taste and see that the LORD is good; blessed is the man who takes refuge in him" (Psalm 34:8). Spiritual "blood work" is essential to spiritual healing and long-term health. When we test ourselves, we'll find "pathogens" or wrong thoughts about God and his purposes. With an accurate diagnosis, we'll be able to apply the right remedy of forgiveness, truth, and hope.

In this book, we'll examine how blood is a showcase of God's marvelous creation and redemption. As we understand the incredible nurturing, cleansing, and healing power he has put into every drop of blood, we'll see the connection between the physical and the spiritual properties of this precious fluid. This study—this "blood work"—will inspire our faith and deepen our sense of wonder at God's care and creativity. Through the limitless creative genius of our awesome God, we will discover that *blood works!* That is my hope for you as you read and study this book.

1

God's Creative Design

" Men go abroad to wonder at the heights of mountains, at the huge waves of the sea, at the long courses of the rivers, at the vast compass of the ocean, at the circular motions of the stars, and they pass by themselves without wondering."

—St. Augustine

To me, telescopes and microscopes are instruments of worship. I look at the incredible expanse of the night sky and realize God simply spoke a word and flung two hundred billion galaxies into space, with about two hundred billion stars in each one. I marvel at the unfathomable power of God, and I realize that I can trust him with my highest hopes and deepest hurts. When I peer into a microscope and look at the incredible intricacy, complexity, and interworking of each cell in the human body, I'm reminded again that God's understanding and care reach into the hidden places in my heart. He knows me intimately—and still loves me deeply.

As a physician, and especially as a hematologist, my study of the human body and the circulatory system reminds me each day of the matchless glory, tender care, and amazing attentiveness of God.

In recent years, the concept of blood in spiritual life has, I'm afraid, fallen out of favor with many people in our churches. They read about the sacrifices in the Old Testament, imagine the scenes, and wince in horror at the gore. They hear about the death of Christ on the cross, and they secretly hope that it was just a big mistake. All that talk about blood seems so, well, barbaric. But I have quite the opposite point of view. I believe that a good understanding of blood in the human body opens our eyes to spiritual insights that can transform our relationships with God and with each other. And when we begin to grasp the true significance of Jesus' blood that was shed to pay for our sins, our hearts are filled with the dual necessities of true spirituality—humility and thankfulness. Far from barbaric, blood is truly beautiful.

Faith and Science

Before we explore the nature of blood as a metaphor of spiritual life, we need to appreciate science as a complement of faith. Too often today, people pit faith against science. They reasonably reject Darwinian theories of unguided evolution, a concept that begins with the presupposition that there is no God, but instead of becoming better students of astronomy, archeology, geology, anatomy, and other important pursuits, they discount science as "sub-Christian" or "anti-Christian." From the outset of this book, I want to disabuse us of this notion. Science isn't an adversary of faith. Properly understood, it opens our minds and hearts to the wonder of God's creative design, and it inspires our faith rather than eroding or threatening it.

Each living cell, even a one-celled animal or plant, is an amazing being. In *Fearfully and Wonderfully Made,* Dr. Paul Brand comments on the wonder of the world not seen by the unaided eye when, as a student, he first looked at an amoeba under a microscope:

"Early one morning, before the laboratory was cluttered with students, I sneaked into the old science building. . . . When I touched one drop of that water to a microscopic slide, a universe came to life. Hundreds of organisms crowded into view. . . . Ah, there it was. An amoeba. Something about the amoeba murmurs that it is one of the most basic and primordial of all creatures. Somehow it has enlisted the everyday forces of millions of spinning atoms so that they now serve life, which differs profoundly from mere matter. Just an oozing bit of gel, the amoeba performs all the basic functions that my body does. It breathes, digests, excretes, reproduces. That busy, throbbing drop gave me my first graphic image of the jungle of life and death we share. I saw the amoeba as an autonomous unit with a fierce urge to live and a stronger urge to propagate itself. It beckoned me on to explore the living cell."[1]

For centuries in the study of history, unbelieving scholars discounted the gospels and Luke's history of the early church in Acts as fairytales. The accounts of miracles by Jesus and the apostles, these historians assumed, were merely fabrications concocted out of thin air centuries later to convince ignorant people that Jesus was God in the flesh. In the past hundred years, however, archeological discoveries have confirmed hundreds of specific references, especially in Luke's detailed accounts, that demonstrate the accuracy of biblical history. The science of archeology strongly supports biblical accounts of history.

---

1   Dr. Paul Brand and Philip Yancey, *Fearfully and Wonderfully Made*, (Zondervan, Grand Rapids, Michigan, 1980), pp. 15-16.

Astronomy also reveals important aspects of the nature of God. The first astronomer, Ptolemy, looked at the night sky and counted 1056 stars. With the magnification of a 1-inch telescope, we can see 225,000 stars; with a 100-inch telescope, we observe 1.5 billion stars; and with a 200-inch telescope, we can see an incredible 1 billion galaxies, each with about 100 billion stars. The Hubble telescope is one of the greatest advances in the history of astronomy. It's named after the astronomer, Edwin Hubble, who, in 1923, discovered that the universe extends past our own galaxy. With the incredible power of its space-based optics, scientists are observing wonders far beyond anything they imagined only a few years before. The optical technology of the Hubble telescope and the absence of earth's atmosphere to cloud its view allow us to see 200 billion galaxies. These numbers quickly become meaningless, so one astronomer put it this way: 100 billion stars in each of 100 billion galaxies (one-fourth of the total of stars now known) is a number similar to the grains of sand on every shore on every beach throughout the entire world! And each of these grains of sand represents an object millions of times larger than our earth.

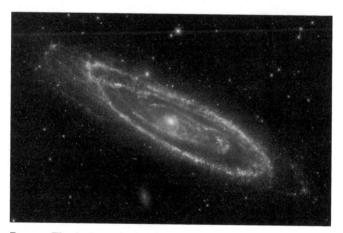

Figure 1. The Andromeda Galaxy.

The diversity of stars in size, variety, and distance from the earth is staggering, but no matter how incredibly immense we find the universe to be, God is far bigger. Isaiah told us that God marked off the heavens "with the breadth of his hand" (Isaiah 40:12), which is the distance between the ends of the little finger and the thumb when the hand is stretched out. This is a poetic way of saying that all of creation is very manageable to our infinite God! He holds it all in his hand.

The human body reveals the genius and complexity of God's design. Subatomic particles, atoms, molecules, and cells perform an intricate dance of power and precision. The body contains between 50 and 75 trillion cells,[2] and each cell is composed of about a trillion atoms. Each cell is a power plant of biofires of hundreds of mitochondria, miniature motors generating adenosine triphosphate, the "molecular unit of currency" of intracellular energy transfer. If we look into each motor, we see tiny wheels turning 100 times each second. The electric fields generated by cells can be even stronger than a high-voltage power line.[3] In addition to supplying energy, mitochondria are involved in signaling, cellular differentiation, the cycle of cell life and death, and cell growth.[4]

Cells in our bodies are born to die—some living only a very short time, but others are capable of surviving for a hundred years. We may think that we don't change much from day to day, but in

---

2   Asimov, Isaac. *The Human Body,* New rev. ed., p. 79; *New Encyclopaedia Britannica,* vol. 6, p. 134; Van Amerogen, C. *The Way Things Work Book of the Body,* p. 13.

3   Campbell, Neil A.; Brad Williamson; Robin J. Heyden, *Biology: Exploring Life,* (2006).

4   McBride HM, Neuspiel M, Wasiak S (2006). "Mitochondria: More Than Just a Powerhouse". *Curr. Biol.* 16.

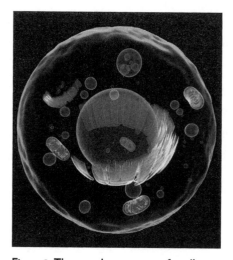

Figure 2. The complex structure of a cell.

a millionth of a second, a trillion atoms in our bodies are replaced, and all of these transitions happen so seamlessly that we don't even notice. The precision and beauty of the way our bodies function is a work of genius. We are incredible machines! Because of God's amazing design, we think, eat, sleep, work, play, exercise, and build relationships with others without the slightest idea of the amazingly complex changes happening each second in our brains, muscles, skeletons, circulation, and organs.

When we look up, we marvel with the psalmist, "The heavens declare the glory of God"; when we look inside, we realize we are "fearfully and wonderfully made." All true science—from archeology to astronomy to human anatomy—stimulates our faith and causes us to marvel at God's attention to every detail. Astrophysicist Hugh Ross commented, "Scientists have identified 109 characteristics of our galaxy and solar system that require exquisite fine-tuning for life's existence and sustenance, and that's to say nothing, yet, about the possibility of organic matter arising from inorganic."[5] American physicist Freeman Dyson commented, "The more I examine the universe and study the details of its architecture, the more evidence I find that the universe in some sense must have known we were

5   Interview with Hugh Ross, "Scientists Are Getting Warmer," *New Man,* September/October 1999, p. 34.

coming."[6] Scottish writer Thomas Carlyle observed, "The universe is but one vast symbol of God."

The problem, of course, is that we're so focused on the things at eye level that we often forget to look up and worship or look down and marvel. With his usual spiritual insight, Thomas Merton observed, "We are living in a world that is absolutely transparent, and God is shining through it all the time. That is not just a fable or a nice story. It is true. If we abandon ourselves to God and forget ourselves, we see it sometimes, and we see it maybe frequently. God shows himself everywhere, in everything—in people, and in things and in nature and in events. It becomes very obvious that God is everywhere and in everything and we cannot be without him. It's impossible. The only thing is that we don't see it."[7] Quite often when I look through a microscope at a slide of a patient's blood, I'm reminded of how marvelous God's creation really is, and too, how fragile we are in a fallen world. My hope is that our study of the amazing properties of blood will open our eyes to the grandeur, beauty, love, and sovereignty of God in us and all around us.

Life is in the Blood

Even in ancient cultures, people understood the importance of blood. God reminded the people of Israel, "The life of every creature is its blood" (Leviticus 17:14). Today, we understand the significance of this truth even more deeply. There are no cells in the human body that can live without continual contact with life-giving blood. Every type of cell, from the ones that survive only moments to those that live for many years, owes its life to the flow of blood. In our

6   Freeman Dyson, *Disturbing the Universe,* (New York, Basic, 1979), p. 250.

7   From "Reflections," *Christianity Today,* January 1999, p. 80.

study, we'll examine three types of cells in human blood: red cells, white cells, and platelets. Each of these performs functions that are essential to life. The red cells nourish every other cell in our bodies with oxygen and other nutrients, and they carry away the toxins our cells create. The role of white cells is surveillance and defense. They are our valiant protectors, continually killing harmful microbes and rushing to the site of any breech in our defenses. Platelets form clots to plug up any breaks in our membranes to stop the bleeding and keep us alive. We'll explore each of these key components in much more detail in subsequent chapters.

Our bodies contain approximately 60,000 miles of blood vessels, branching innumerable times from the aorta to the smallest capillaries that touch each cell. Through this delivery system, blood provides everything our cells need to live, and they take away waste that would poison us. At the cellular level, capillaries are so small that they are about the size of a single red blood cell, and in fact, red cells sometimes have to perform distortions to get through the small openings. The walls of the capillaries are thin and porous to allow for the exchange of molecules, such as oxygen, water, sugar, electrolytes, carbon dioxide, and certain proteins.

To connect with all the cells in the body, capillary walls cover an area of about 70,000 square feet. The walls are so delicate that they rupture under the tension of one three-thousandths of the force needed to tear toilet tissue.[8] Ruptures allow blood cells to escape, resulting in bruising.

The circulatory system is the epitome of consistency. Every day, the heart beats 100,000 times, and over an average lifespan, this amazing machine beats 2.5 billion times, pumping 60 million

---

8   John R. Cameron, James G. Skofronick, and Roderick M. Grant, *Physics of the Body*, (Madison, WI: Medical Physics Publishing, 1999), p. 191.

gallons of blood. During this time, the heart never takes time off. We can't afford for it to take a break—even a few minutes without blood supply causes severe brain damage or death.

Virtually all other cells in the human body are stationary, but blood is mobile tissue, carrying nutrients to every part of the body—parts we see and parts most of us don't even know exist—protecting us from harm, healing our wounds, and eliminating toxins that threaten to harm us.

The Implications and Impact of Blood

American essayist and poet Ralph Waldo Emerson observed, "What lies before us and what lies behind us are small matters compared to what lies within us. And when we bring what is within us out into the world, miracles happen." In our examination of blood, I want to bring the wonders within us out into the world to showcase God's masterpiece of creation and redemption. In fact, the implications of blood fall into two areas: common grace and saving grace.

Common grace

Common grace is God's kindness and provision for every person on the planet, without distinction between believers and unbelievers. Creation itself is a mark of common grace. The beautiful structures of the body, the seasons, crops and cattle that provide sustenance for every person in every culture, gravity to keep us grounded so we don't float off into space, the relationships of families, government to enact laws to protect us, and conscience, the ingrained sense of right and wrong, are gifts to every human life.

Paul explained God's common grace to the Colossians when he wrote, "For by [Christ] all things were created: things in heaven and on earth, visible and invisible, whether thrones or powers or rulers or authorities; all things were created by him and for him. He is before all things, and in him all things hold together" (Colossians 1:16-17). And in his most powerful theological treatise, the letter to the Christians in Rome, Paul told them that the government is "a minister of God" (Romans 13:6) to provide order and safety for its citizens. Jesus told us that the cycles of nature provide for all of us. He said, "Your Father in heaven . . . causes his sun to rise on the evil and the good, and sends rain on the righteous and the unrighteous" (Matthew 5:46).

In a beautiful devotional poem in Psalm 139, David reflected on the power and creativity of God. He marveled that God knows everything we say and do, "even before a word is on my tongue," and he is amazed that God is ubiquitous—everywhere in the universe at once. When he thought about his own body's intricate design, he realized that God had "knit" him together when he was in his mother's womb. The complexity of the human body elicited both awe and wonder. David marveled,

"For you created my inmost being;
    you knit me together in my mother's womb.
I praise you because I am fearfully and wonderfully made;
    your works are wonderful,
    I know that full well.
My frame was not hidden from you
    when I was made in the secret place.
    When I was woven together in the depths of the earth. . . .
How precious to me are your thoughts, O God!
    How vast is the sum of them!" (Psalm 139:13-15, 17).

I believe scientists and doctors have a distinct advantage in noticing common grace all around us. As we explore space, plastics, nanotechnology, the meticulous working of human anatomy, and countless other studies, we come face to face with the marvelous mechanisms God has created to make our lives work so well. We've discovered a lot, but we're on the leading edge of far more discoveries. Every year, we uncover new insights and explore new ways to make life even better, based on God's provision of life, food, shelter, reason, electromagnetism, and all the other systems he has instituted for every person on earth to enjoy.

The discoveries we've made in the field of hematology in the past decade have given us a clearer understanding of the amazing design and interworking of each aspect of human blood. As we increasingly understand these beautiful complexities, we can prevent and treat diseases related to the *hematopoietic* (blood forming) system. For example, in the last several years, we have made great strides in treating multiple myeloma (MM), cancer of the plasma in bone marrow. In a person with this disease, abnormal plasma cells (or myeloma cells) multiply, resulting in reduced blood production, which in turn leads to anemia and fatigue. Bone damage from the disease may also cause painful rib and spinal-compression fractures. Researchers have characterized a precursor condition (monoclonal gammopathy), identifying factors that predict the course of the disease. With these advances, they have developed new systems for classifying the disease. Today, there is far more hope for these patients than ever before. Research, motivated in part by the pandemic of HIV, has opened new avenues of understanding of the intricate structure and interworkings of T and B lymphocytes. We now have more understanding so we can more effectively treat childhood leukemias and other white blood cell cancers, greatly increasing survival and cure rates.

We enjoy so many blessings, especially in Western culture, that we forget what life would be like if any of the benefits of common grace were altered even by a fraction. By God's gracious design, we enjoy a measure of protection and provision that makes life possible, and indeed, pleasurable, for billions of people. Even the solutions to some of the world's most intractable problems aren't mysterious. Though millions die from malaria each year in the tropics, a 35-cent dose of medicine would prevent the disease. God's grace is common to all of us, but he has given us the privilege and responsibility to use it to help others. Bible scholar Louis Berkhof observed, "[Common grace] curbs the destructive power of sin, maintains in a measure the moral order of the universe, thus making an orderly life possible, distributes in varying degrees gifts and talents among men, promotes the development of science and art, and showers untold blessings upon the children of men."[9]

Our blood is one of the most powerful examples of common grace in our lives, and it tells us volumes about God's tender, tenacious care to provide for our every need (including those we don't even know about), remove poisons, protect us, and heal our hurts. We are God's masterpiece, the pinnacle of his creative design. Our bodies, both in structure (anatomy) and function (physiology), proclaim the majesty of God. As we look at God's marvelous design reflected in the nature of our blood, we'll be inspired to worship him for his creativity, power, and precision. As we look at the wonder of our blood, we'll see it as a metaphor of the second kind of grace God gives us: special or saving grace.

Saving grace

The crucial importance of blood is woven throughout the Bible. From Genesis to Revelation, the writers tell us that life itself—both

---

9   Louis Berkhof, *Systematic Theology*, 4th ed. (Grand Rapids: Eerdmans, 1979), p. 434.

physical and spiritual—is found in this precious fluid. The Bible doesn't always use the exact term of "blood" to communicate the message of the price paid for forgiveness. Sometimes, it uses "death," "sacrifice," "payment," "redemption," "atonement," "substitution," "propitiation," "justification," or other words, but they all refer to a price paid for the forgiveness of sins and the restoration of a relationship with God. Some scholars say that the concept of a blood sacrifice is either explicit or implicit in every passage throughout the entire biblical record.

When the Bible says, "Life is in the blood," it carries the dual meaning of life and death. Even in ancient times, people understood that people and other types of animals couldn't live without the flow of life-giving blood. They didn't understand all the properties we understand now, and in fact, it wasn't until Dutch scientist Antoni van Leeuwenhoek looked through a microscope in the 17th century that scientists understood that there were different types of cells in our blood. The ancient people of the Bible, however, lived agrarian lives, and they were closer to the realities of life than most people alive today, especially Westerners. Instead of picking up shrink-wrapped steaks at the grocery store, they slaughtered the animals they ate. To them, the sight of blood was a common phenomenon.

From the beginning, God instituted blood sacrifice as an offering for sin. In the Old Testament sacrificial system, priests and individuals slit the throats of animals—choice, costly, unblemished animals—to offer to God to pay for sin. The act of killing the animal and watching the blood flow from its neck until it died is a graphic depiction of two important lessons: sin is so serious that something (or Someone) has to die to pay for it, and the one who offers the sacrifice pays a high price for forgiveness. In the first family, two brothers tried different methods to pay for their sins and establish a connection with God. The Scriptures tell us, "Now Abel kept flocks, and Cain worked the soil. In the course of time Cain brought some of the fruits of the soil as an offering to the LORD. But Abel brought fat portions from some of the firstborn of his flock. The LORD looked with favor on Abel and his offering, but on Cain and his offering he did not look with favor" (Genesis 4:2-5). God must have made it clear to both brothers that he expected a blood sacrifice, but only one was willing to pay the high price.

In the Pentateuch, the first five books of the Bible, God gives detailed instructions about how people and priests were to offer sacrifices and handle blood with the utmost respect. For instance, we read in Deuteronomy, "If an animal has a defect, is lame or blind, or has any serious flaw, you must not sacrifice it to the LORD your God. You are to eat it in your own towns. Both the ceremonially unclean and the clean may eat it, as if it were gazelle or deer. But you must not eat the blood; pour it out on the ground like water" (Deuteronomy 15:21-23). Sin is serious business. In our culture, many of us are entertained by sins depicted on television every night, we wink when we hear about adultery, and we take it for granted that lies are part of every business deal. But God doesn't see it that way. Sin is anything that falls short of the glory, truth, and love of God—and anything we love more than him. It rips the fabric of God's intentions for our relationship with him and with those around us. Sin poisons our own hearts and hurts those we say we love. But it's not just about breaking "the Big Ten." It's much more important than that. When we sin, we not only break one of God's rules; we break his heart.

To show how grave sin really is, God instituted a covenant with his people based on animal sacrifice. To experience forgiveness, blood had to be spilled and a harmless animal had to die. Every time an animal was killed on the altar, the person received a graphic reminder that sin is tragic and forgiveness is costly. Sometimes, people tried to offer animals they didn't value, ones that wouldn't have been sold in the meat market because the animals were flawed. They assumed God wouldn't notice, but he did. Through the prophet Malachi, God accused the people, "When you bring blind animals for sacrifice, is that not wrong? When you sacrifice crippled or diseased animals, is that not wrong? Try offering them to your governor! Would he be pleased with you? Would he accept you?" (Malachi 1:8) If their governor wouldn't accept the animal, why would they think that Almighty God, the creator of the universe, would accept a blind, crippled, or diseased offering? No, God requires the best sacrifice we can offer. The perfect lambs offered by the priests at the temple were only a shadow of the Lamb of God who would someday come to offer himself as the ultimate sacrifice for the sins of the world.

The death of Christ deals with our past, our present, and our future. It provides the necessary atonement for all our sins—not parts of them or some of them. Because of him, we're free today, not free to sin, but free to live for the one who loves us and gave himself for us. And it offers the most glowing, magnificent promise ever given: that you and I will be with him in glory for all time because we've been washed in the blood of the Lamb.

We can't fully appreciate the death of Christ until we realize that he died in our place. Our sins deserve death, and they require death as a payment. Jesus shed his blood as a substitute for the payment we owed but could never pay. When we say we've been "redeemed," it means that Someone has paid the price to set us free. During the Civil War, civilians suffered terribly in the states of Missouri and Kansas. A renegade group of Southern sympathizers called Quantrill's Raiders burned and looted Lawrence, Kansas, murdering innocent people.

Men in Kansas formed a militia to protect their homes and families. They saw Quantrill's men as criminals, not soldiers, and they had orders to execute any they captured. Soon, the militia surrounded a group of raiders, and they lined them up in front of a firing squad. Suddenly, a man ran out of the woods shouting, "Wait! Don't shoot!" He pointed to one of the men to be shot, and he told the militia commander, "Let that man go free. He has a wife and four children, and he's needed at home. Let me take his place."

The commander considered this unusual appeal, and he decided to grant the man's wish. They released the captured raider and put the other man in his place. When the shots were fired, he fell dead, and the other man went home. Later, he came back to the scene, uncovered his substitute's body, and carried it to a cemetery for proper burial. Above the grave, he erected a headstone that read, "He took my place. He died for me."

Jesus said, "Greater love has no one than this, that he lay down his life for his friends" (John 15:13). In the same way this man sacrificed himself for his friend, Jesus put himself in our place and paid the awful penalty we can't afford to pay.

Christ's payment on the cross is both judicial and relational. The Scriptures paint the picture of a courtroom where the guilty (that's you and me) stand trial before the Judge of All. The prosecutor is Satan, the accuser of the brethren, and our defense counsel is Jesus Christ. We are, there's no doubt, guilty as charged of a long list of crimes of selfishness. We deserve the sentence of death, but our Advocate steps out and pays the full price on our behalf. We deserve to go to the firing squad, but he stands in our place and takes our capital punishment so that we can go free. When we begin to grasp this incredible fact, our hearts soar and sing with gratitude, and we look for every way possible to honor the One who loves us so much.

Paul explained the connection between the death of Christ and glad obedience when he wrote to the Corinthians, "For Christ's love compels us, because we are convinced that one died for all, and therefore all died. And he died for all, that those who live should no longer live for themselves but for him who died for them and was raised again" (2 Corinthians 5:14-15). A fuller grasp of the importance of blood in our spiritual life causes us to view sin more seriously, but at the same time, we appreciate God's wonderful forgiveness more than ever before. We'll love him more, long to please him with all our hearts, and obey him—not because we feel forced to, but because we genuinely want to.

Blood and Purpose

The gospel of Jesus Christ is centered on the most important events in history: his death and resurrection. His blood paid set us free, and his resurrection promises new life—now and forever. We all have many different ways we identify ourselves. I'm a husband, father, friend, mediocre golfer, pastor, and doctor. But the description in a biographical sketch or words on a nametag pale in comparison with the most important factor in my identity: I've been ransomed from sin, spiritual death, and hell by Jesus Christ, and now I belong to him. When the believers in Corinth had drifted away from Jesus, Paul reminded them, "Do you not know that your body is a temple of the Holy Spirit, who is in you, whom you have received from God? You are not your own; you were bought at a price. Therefore honor God with your body" (1 Corinthians 6:19-20).

What does it mean that we've been bought by the blood of Christ? It changes our attitudes, our destiny, and our purpose in this life. Many of the things that used to seem so important to us now appear quite trivial, and the things of God that used to bore us or annoy us now take first place in our lives. We realize that the value of a human soul—ours or anyone else's—is worth more than anything else in the world. Jesus told his followers, "If anyone would come after me, he must deny himself and take up his cross and follow me. For whoever wants to save his life will lose it, but whoever loses his life for me will find it. What good will it be for a man if he gains the whole world, yet forfeits his soul? Or what can a man give in exchange for his soul?" (Matthew 16:24-26) This means that if we put all the world's wealth—all the gold, oil, real estate, diamonds, cars, cash, and everything else of value—on one side of a scale, and we put the most obscure person in the world—or maybe you or me—on the other, the balance would tip toward the one soul because that person is worth more than everything else. The blood of Jesus is the only thing that can give life to a dead heart, and he has given us life by dying in our place. Even if you or I were the only people who ever lived, Jesus would have stepped out of heaven to die for us. His death wasn't a tragic accident or a colossal misunderstanding, and he wasn't coerced. He chose to give his life as a ransom for many. He was more than willing to suffer and die for you and me.

Because we've been bought with the blood of Jesus, we belong to him, and he gives us the privilege of living for him each day. Because of him, our lives have eternal purpose! The meaning in our lives doesn't come from having one more possession or getting promoted one more rung up the corporate ladder. It comes from knowing that our lives really matter in God's kingdom. In his insightful book, *The Call*, Os Guinness defines our spiritual calling as "the truth that God calls us to himself so decisively that everything we are, everything we do, and everything we have is invested with a special devotion and dynamism lived out as a response to his summons and service."[10] Our purpose, our sense of calling, is not primarily to a career or a type of service, or to a company or a particular church. It is first and foremost to God himself. The impact of that relationship shapes every fiber of our being, determines every action we do, and gives direction to how we use every resource we have.

The analogy of the body applies directly to our relationships in the family of God. Paul said that the church is "the body of Christ." When toxins of bitterness and jealousy aren't removed by the forgiveness of Christ, we experience heartache and headaches in our relationships with each other. But if each of us, like cells in the body, is being nourished, protected, and healed by one another as we impart life-giving love, forgiveness, and truth to each other, we grow strong and make a difference in our community and the wider world.

Some of the most beautiful songs written in church history describe the wonder of Christ's precious blood. They do much more than articulate the event of the cross; they help us grasp the spiritual power of the cross to change our lives. I want to include one of these hymns in every chapter of the book. Please don't skip over these. Take time to read them slowly and make the words your own. One of my favorites is "At the Cross" by Isaac Watts:

"Alas! and did my Savior bleed

And did my Sov'reign die?

Would He devote that sacred head

For such a worm as I?

---

10 Os Guinness, *The Call*, (Word Publishing, Nashville, 1998), p. 4.

Refrain:

At the cross, at the cross where I first saw the light,

And the burden of my heart rolled away,

It was there by faith I received my sight,

And now I am happy all the day!

Thy body slain, sweet Jesus, Thine—

And bathed in its own blood—

While the firm mark of wrath divine,

His soul in anguish stood.

Was it for crimes that I had done

He groaned upon the tree?

Amazing pity! grace unknown!

And love beyond degree!

Well might the sun in darkness hide

And shut his glories in,

When Christ, the mighty Maker died,

For man the creature's sin.

Thus might I hide my blushing face

While His dear cross appears,

Dissolve my heart in thankfulness,

And melt my eyes to tears.

But drops of grief can ne'er repay
The debt of love I owe:
Here, Lord, I give myself away,
Tis all that I can do." [11]

My Promise to You

I hope that God uses the concepts and stories in this book to amplify your faith and your love for God. As you see how God uses blood to impart both common grace and saving grace, you'll have a deeper appreciation for the majesty and tender care of God. You'll marvel at the intricacies of the human body, and particularly the blood, and you'll have a richer, deeper appreciation for the high cost Jesus paid to rescue you from sin, hell, and death.

The message of the cross invites us to be sober about our sins, but it frees our hearts to love him and enjoy him like never before. The extreme payment of the Savior's death tells us how much God loves us, and it clears away barriers in our relationships with one another. We may look different on the outside—we may have different skin colors, speak in different languages, have different customs, and live in different parts of the world—but blood is the same the world over. When someone needs a transfusion or an organ transplant, he doesn't care about the differences any more. In the same way, when we've experienced a transfusion of the forgiveness of God and the transplant of his nature into our hearts, we don't care about the differences in the members of his family. We learn to overlook our differences and see our commonalities.

---

11 "At the Cross," by Isaac Watts, published in 1707.

I've included some questions at the end of each chapter to help you think more deeply about the principles and applications. You may want to use the book in a small group or class to encourage each other.

Think about it...

1. Before reading this chapter, did you see blood in the Bible as barbaric or beautiful? Explain your answer.

2. When was the last time you looked through a telescope or microscope? Did it inspire a sense of amazement? Explain your answer.

3. What are some evidences of God's common grace in your life? Why don't we think about them more than we do? What difference would it make if we reflected about them more?

4. Why is a sense of wonder important to our faith? What happens to our relationship with God if we don't have this sense of wonder?

5. What do you hope to get out of this book?

Red Cells:
The Cycle of Life

" There is no language more universal nor more ancient.

From time immemorial, people from every culture of the

world have used the blood to speak those unutterable

feelings of the soul which all of us know. As such, it is a

common ingredient of man's aspiration beyond himself."

—Robert Coleman

When van Leeuwenhoek looked at blood under his microscope centuries ago, he discovered countless red cells, the most numerous cells in our blood. Also called *erythrocytes*, they perform a vital function of taking nourishment to every cell in the body and carrying away harmful toxins. Red cells are the only cell in the body without a nucleus, but they have an iron-rich molecule called *hemoglobin*, which combines with oxygen. The red cells then serve as billions of taxis, transporting oxygen and other nutrients through the arteries and into the capillaries to every cell in the body. The cycle of life is completed when the oxygen-depleted red cell picks up a new passenger, carbon dioxide, to carry it to the lungs to be exhaled. No cell can live without this vital exchange.

Every Breath

The transportation of oxygen begins in the lungs. With every breath, we inhale trillions of oxygen molecules. In fact, in every breath, we absorb 150 million molecules breathed by Jesus Christ.[12] Like the blood vessels, the airways in the lungs branch into smaller and smaller tubes, ultimately forming alveoli, with incredibly thin membranes that allow the penetration of gas molecules. The exchange of gases, oxygen and carbon dioxide, occurs by diffusion. The pressure of oxygen in the alveoli must be kept at a higher level than the pressure in the blood, and the pressure of carbon dioxide in the alveoli must be kept at a lower lever than in the blood. The difference in pressure forces oxygen into the blood and forces carbon dioxide out. We perform this function, breathing, about 20,000 times a day.

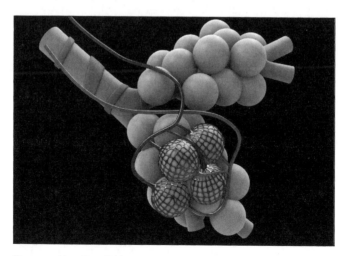

Figure 3. Alveoli in the lungs.

12 Cameron, et al, p. 146.

When we eat, the digestive system breaks down the food into sugars and proteins, and eventually, the red cells carry these, along with the oxygen, to the cells throughout our bodies.

Red cells, which look like small red donuts, live 120 days. Each drop of human blood contains over 5 million red cells. Every second, 8 million of them die, but each second, 8 million more are produced. In an average lifetime, a person's red cells arranged in single file would reach from the earth to the sun and back five times! At any given time, the single file of red cells in a person's body would extend around the equator four times.

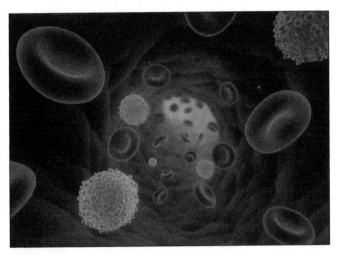

Figure 4. Blood streaming through a vessel.

In the red cells, each hemoglobin molecule can carry millions of oxygen atoms to replenish the energy-starved cells in the body along the path of the vessels and capillaries. Each cell in our bodies depends on the continuous supply of oxygen and other nutrients, and some, like our brains, experience severe problems if they are deprived of oxygen for even a few minutes.

The body can't function properly without the elimination of toxins from the cells. Left to accumulate, these toxins would soon poison our bodies and we would die.

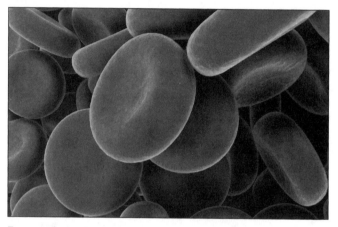

Figure 5. Red cells.

One of the most dramatic demonstrations of the necessity to eliminate toxins occurred on the fabled and flawed flight of Apollo 13. After the oxygen tank exploded, the astronauts on the way to the moon looked at their monitors and realized the level of carbon dioxide was rising too far and too fast. In a Herculean effort by the engineers of the ground crew at NASA in Houston, a solution was finally found, and improvised "scrubbers" eliminated carbon dioxide from the air in the space capsule. As the movie depicted, the margin of life and death was slim. If they hadn't found the solution quickly, the men would have died. High levels of carbon dioxide in the capsule and in our cells aren't just nuisances; they kill. Sleep apnea and chronic obstructive pulmonary disease (COPD) are two disorders that threaten people because they allow carbon dioxide to build up. Other organs, such as the liver and kidney, eliminate other toxins from the body, and they use the blood as a transportation system to carry these toxins to be eliminated.

Anemia, the most common blood disorder, is directly related to red cells. The term covers a wide range of differing problems, but generally, it refers to excessive blood loss (such as through hemorrhage) or a decrease in the body's production of red cells in the bone marrow. It leads to hypoxia, the lack of oxygen getting to the body's cells. Without a fully functioning cycle of life in the red cells, people experience a wide range of symptoms, including feelings of weakness, the inability to concentrate, shortness of breath upon exertion, and in severe cases, heart palpitations as the heart tries to compensate for the body's lack of oxygen by pumping more vigorously.

Red Cells and the Blood of Christ

Christ's sacrifice for us gives us the nourishment of love and eliminates the toxin of sin. Like oxygen from red cells replenishing starved, carbon dioxide laden tissues, we soak up his love and power, and if we realize how much we desperately need him, we long for his kindness, grace, and strength like a depleted cell waits for the hemoglobin to release oxygen and nutrients to keep it alive. Before Jesus was betrayed, he ate a final meal with his disciples. John, who was there, tells us, "It was just before the Passover Feast. Jesus knew that the time had come for him to leave this world and go to the Father. Having loved his own who were in the world, he now showed them the full extent of his love" (John 13:1). In the gospels, "the time" always refers to Jesus' impending death. Before that night, he had told his mother at a wedding and his brothers before a feast that his time had not yet come. But now, the moment had arrived that all of history had anticipated. God himself would die to pay for the sins of the world. "T'is mystery all! The immortal dies!" It was the supreme demonstration of love.

The nourishment of love and power

Throughout the accounts of the gospel writers, we realize that Jesus turned everything upside down. The "insiders," who thought they were shoe-ins for God's kingdom because they were so meticulous in keeping the laws, became outsiders because they refused to embrace Jesus as the Messiah. But the "outsiders" of their society—prostitutes, tax gatherers, adulterers, the poor, the blind, the lame, the sick, lepers, and women—were attracted to his tenderness and gracious acceptance. The death of Jesus is the most marvelous demonstration of soul-nourishing love the world has ever known, but there has to be a pressure gradient: we have to realize our desperate need for him so that we receive him and benefit from his grace. Without a compelling sense of need, we keep our hearts walled off and let him pass by.

Christ also nourishes us with his power. When we trust in him, his Spirit comes to live inside us, filling our hearts with hope and strength so that we overflow in gratitude and desire to please him. At the Feast of Booths in Jerusalem, each day's sacrifices increased in importance to a crescendo on the last day. John explains, "On the last and greatest day of the Feast, Jesus stood and said in a loud voice, 'If anyone is thirsty, let him come to me and drink. Whoever believes in me, as the Scripture has said, streams of living water will flow from within him.' By this he meant the Spirit, whom those who believed in him were later to receive" (John 7:37-39).

How powerful is the Spirit in us? Paul tells us that the Spirit's strength in us is nothing less than the same power that raised Jesus from the tomb! In his prayer for the Christians in Ephesus, he wrote,

"That power is like the working of his mighty strength, which he exerted in Christ when he raised him from the dead and seated him at his right hand in the heavenly realms, far above all rule and authority, power and dominion, and every title that can be given, not only in the present age but also in the one to come" (Ephesians 1:19-21). That's the power God has put into us the moment we were born again. To experience this strength, we don't need any more of him, but perhaps he needs more from us.

In the Christian life, we don't begin the first day by trusting in Jesus and then gut it out on our own from then on. No, like the red cells continually feeding every cell in our bodies, we depend on God every second of every day for life, peace, strength, joy, and love. Without his love and power feeding our hearts like hemoglobin continuously releasing oxygen to our cells, we become spiritually and emotionally anemic. For us, the symptoms are dramatic and painful. We trust in our own wisdom and power to make life work, and we fail miserably. We may be outwardly successful, but our hearts atrophy and become self-righteous, discouraged, or complacent. And without the constant exchange of spiritual nutrients and toxins, we experience the death of our God-given sense of purpose.

Sin as life's toxin

Sin is the noxious poison in our lives that has to be eliminated if we're going to survive and thrive. In our modern age of political correctness, we tolerate sin in our lives and excuse it in others. Without a genuine grasp of the destructive nature of sinful attitudes and actions, we lose our way spiritually. We fail to appreciate the richness of God's forgiveness and devalue his majesty and greatness. Without his constant supply of love and forgiveness, our souls atrophy. We become zombies, the living dead, going through the motions of life but without joy, love, excitement, and wonder. When God warned Adam and Eve to avoid eating fruit from a single tree in the Garden, he said, "On the day you eat of it, you will surely die" (Genesis 2:17). Some people would say, "Well, God was wrong. They didn't die after all." But they did. Their bodies began the process of dying, and their souls were cut off from the beauty, kindness, and strength of God. Physical death came later, but they experienced spiritual death at that instant.

Like Adam and Eve, many people around us today look alive on the outside, but they're dead on the inside. Sin poisons families and communities as well as individuals. When we see news reports of hatred, bigotry, abuse, and violence, we're seeing the necrotic effects of sin on our culture. When we see so many people hungry and without medical supplies while countless others live in luxury, we get a glimpse of the spiritual death that values personal riches and devalues the lives of the poor. I've traveled to parts of Africa where many people, especially young children, died from water-borne diseases because of unsanitary water, but when the church dug a well and provided fresh drinking water, the infection and death rates were cut in half. How many other villages need us to overcome spiritual death and come to life so that we care enough to help them?

Theologians talk about two aspects of God: his *transcendence*, he is "far above all," and his *immanence*, he is "closer than our breath." In our culture, we've swung the pendulum far to the side of immanence, making God our "Buddy" and "the Man Upstairs." We've made God common and approachable, but at the expense of his holiness and majesty. We don't need to discard either one, but hold them both in our two hands. When we treat God as a Cosmic Friend, we devalue everything about him, his greatness and grace, and we discount the significance of sin that separates unbelievers from him and dishonors him in the lives of those who claim to know him. Instead of worshipping him and bowing in awe, we demand that he jump through our hoops and give us what we want. A few years ago, Charles J. Sykes wrote a piercing book about our culture called *A Nation of Victims*. In it, he described how our society has shifted from taking responsibility to demanding that others (parents, teachers, government, and God) meet all our needs—and meet them quickly. People who see themselves as victims don't believe they need to be forgiven, and they sure aren't willing to forgive those who disappoint them. The sin we experience in our culture and in our private lives today isn't just saying a bad word here and there or being a little bit selfish; it's a terribly perverse view of the nature of God and our place in his universe, and it leads to a tragic erosion of personal responsibility.

Sin is powerful and destructive. It pollutes our motives, ruins our relationships, and distorts our sense of purpose. Jesus warned, "The thief comes only to steal and kill and destroy; I have come that they may have life, and have it to the full" (John 10:10). God wants us to know him, love him, and follow him in the greatest adventure life can offer, but the enemy of our souls is a thief who wants to rob us of God's wonderful purposes, kill our hearts, and destroy the beautiful things God wants to do in and through us. When we realize the destructive nature of sin, we'll take it much more seriously.

Those of us who tolerate sin have little appreciation or experience of forgiveness. When we blow it and hurt others and ourselves, we quickly say things like, "I couldn't help it," "It's not that bad," "It didn't even happen," or "What's the big deal? Everybody's doing it." When Adam and Eve sinned, their instant response was to cover themselves, hide from God, and blame each other for their problems. (Adam also blamed God!) We haven't altered our pattern much in the years since that day.

Being honest about our faults and flaws is the first step, but it's one that is often hard to take. In the spring, King David should have gone out to battle with his army, but he stayed behind in Jerusalem. One day, he walked out on his balcony and saw a beautiful woman on a rooftop below. His lust for her led him to commit adultery and then conspire with his army commander to have her husband killed in battle. But it wasn't a military casualty—it was murder. For a long time, David tried to act like he had done nothing wrong. Finally, his friend Nathan confronted him, and he admitted his sin. During the time of spiritual silence, David died a thousand deaths as his sin poisoned his heart. In a psalm he wrote to describe his experience with shame and guilt (the natural consequences of letting the toxin of sin infect us), David wrote,

> *"When I kept silent,*
>
> > *my bones wasted away*
> >
> > *through my groaning all day long.*
>
> *For day and night*
>
> > *your hand was heavy upon me;*
> >
> > *my strength was sapped*
> >
> > *as in the heat of summer"* (Psalm 32:3-4).

As long as he let the poison of sin affect him, David suffered physical weakness and spiritual anemia. He felt weak, sick, and helpless. But God's forgiveness is always present if we'll just embrace it. Finally, David took God's hand:

> *"Then I acknowledged my sin to you*
>
> > *and did not cover up my iniquity.*
>
> *I said, 'I will confess*

my transgressions to the LORD'—
and you forgave
the guilt of my sin.
You are my hiding place;
you will protect me from trouble
and surround me with songs of deliverance"
(Psalm 32:5,7).

David and other prophets in the Old Testament looked forward to the ultimate sacrifice for sin: Jesus the Messiah. They knew that when he came, there would be no more need for animals to be killed to pay for sins because the Son of God's blood was more than enough to forgive every sin of every person who ever lived. Today, we look back at the death of Christ and the shedding of his blood to rid our hearts of the poison of sin, and our hearts sing with gratitude. Robert Lowry captured this sentiment when he wrote the classic, "Nothing But the Blood of Jesus":

"What can wash away my sin?
Nothing but the blood of Jesus;
What can make me whole again?
Nothing but the blood of Jesus.

Oh! precious is the flow
That makes me white as snow;
No other fount I know,
Nothing but the blood of Jesus.

For my cleansing this I see—
Nothing but the blood of Jesus!
For my pardon this my plea—
Nothing but the blood of Jesus!" [13]

Two mistakes

People often make one of two mistakes when they think about the gospel message of Christ's sacrifice of blood to redeem us. They are either romantic existentialists or religious moralists.

Existentialists live by their feelings, and they believe they deserve for God to give them a happy, prosperous life. Like the younger brother in the parable of the prodigal son, they want what they want, and they want it now! The expectation of immediate gratification has crept into a few corners of the church. Some preachers proclaim a "prosperity gospel," claiming that God's chief purpose is to make his children happy and wealthy. People who buy what these preachers are selling have incredibly high expectations, and in fact, unrealistic expectations of God, and they become deeply disillusioned when God doesn't dance to their tune. The blood of Jesus promises us many things, but not health and wealth. It guarantees us entrance into the kingdom, and it provides peace during times of heartache and confusion. Jesus promises his presence in the midst of struggles, but he never promises the elimination of those struggles. Quite the opposite. He said, "In this world you will have trouble. But take heart! I have overcome the world" (John 16:33). When a man announced his loyalty to him, Jesus quickly saw that the man was an existentialist, and he needed a dose of reality. The man promised

---

13 "Nothing But the Blood of Jesus," words and music by Robert Lowry, 1876.

naively, "I will follow you wherever you go." Jesus replied, "Foxes have holes and birds of the air have nests, but the Son of Man has no place to lay his head" (Luke 9:57-58). Jesus always asks us to count the cost.

An accurate understanding of the sacrifice of Christ helps us look beyond any idealistic pretensions and grasp both the beauty and the challenge of following the Savior. Forgiveness is a magnificent gift, but when we embrace it, we turn over our lives to the care and direction of a loving, wise, and unpredictable King. We are no longer our own, we've been bought with a price, and we shouldn't expect to have more blessings and prosperity than our master had when he was on earth. We're not above our teacher. C. S. Lewis' *The Chronicles of Narnia* are full of spiritual insights. Early in the first book of the series, *The Lion, the Witch, and the Wardrobe*, Mrs. Beaver tells Lucy about Aslan, the great lion of Narnia, who is a Christ-figure in the stories. Mrs. Beaver tells the little girl of Aslan's power and majesty, and how he sometimes appears in times of trouble. Then Lucy, overwhelmed with the thought that she might someday actually face this awesome beast, asks timidly, "Is he safe?"

"Oh no, dearie," Mrs. Beaver almost laughs at the thought. "He's not safe. But he's good."

If we don't have some sense that following Christ is the most thrilling and threatening adventure the world has ever known, it may not be Christ that we're following.

The second error, the mistake of religious moralism, is a very different problem. Some of us begin our Christian lives by trusting Christ's sacrifice for our sins, but poor teaching, bad models, or indwelling sin causes us to think we can now earn God's approval by doing enough right things. We live by the law, feeling powerful and righteous because we've done this or that good deed, and we've avoided this or that sin, so we can puff out our chests and prove that we're acceptable. The elder brother in Jesus' story of the prodigal son made this mistake. When his father invited him to join the celebration because his wayward brother had repented and come home, the elder brother barked, "Look! All these years I've been slaving for you and never disobeyed your orders. Yet you never gave me even a young goat so I could celebrate with my friends. But when this son of yours who has squandered your property with prostitutes comes home, you kill the fattened calf for him!" (Luke 15:29-30)

Can you feel the elder brother's resentment? He said he'd been "slaving" all these years, doing all the right things but for all the wrong reasons. He insisted that he had "never disobeyed" his father. He had set the bar high, and he had achieved it! But his rigid rule keeping filled him with bitterness. He hated the fact that his dad was spending lavishly on a party for his brother. The elder brother is much like many people in our churches today. They have forgotten the marvelous freedom and joy that comes when we remember Christ's sacrifice for us. Keeping rules looks pious, but it leaves our hearts empty. To fill them, we look at others who aren't keeping the rules quite as well, and we feel superior. We delight in finding specs in their eyes, but we don't see the logs in our own.

Resentment and self-righteousness are the byproducts of comparison. To illustrate the damage done by moralistic rule keeping, Jesus told a story of a hated tax collector and a rule keeping Pharisee going to the temple to pray. He said, "Two men went up to the temple to pray, one a Pharisee and the other a tax collector. The Pharisee stood up and prayed about himself: 'God, I thank you that I am not like other men—robbers, evildoers, adulterers—or even like this tax collector. I fast twice a week and give a tenth of all I get' " (Luke 18:10-12).

Tax collectors weren't like our IRS agents. They were traitors. They were Jews who collaborated with the Romans to extort extra taxes from their own people. They were the most hated people in the land. It was easy for a Pharisee, who kept hundreds of extra laws every week in addition to the laws of the Bible, to feel superior to a despised tax collector. But the parable doesn't end here. Jesus said that a few feet away, the tax collector looked down in shame and beat his chest. He pleaded, "God, have mercy on me, a sinner" (Luke 18:13).

To the astonishment of the people listening to Jesus that day, he concluded, "I tell you that this man [the repentant tax collector], rather than the other, went home justified before God. For everyone who exalts himself will be humbled, and he who humbles himself will be exalted" (Luke 18:14).

Another way

The gospel of Christ offers a third alternative to romantic existentialism and religious moralism. When we look at the blood Jesus spilled for us, we realize that neither of those ways deals with our deepest needs or fulfills our highest hopes. The sacrifice of Jesus doesn't minimize our sins—it looks them squarely in the eye and says, "I paid the price. You're forgiven." And it doesn't let us think we can impress God by keeping a set of rules. It says, "There's no one righteous. No not one, but I forgive you without reservation." The gospel invites us to be completely honest about our secret sins because we have the promise of being fully forgiven, completely loved, and totally accepted by God through Christ. Jesus doesn't excuse our sins. He doesn't say they don't matter. He never looks the other way and denies they even exist. He took them onto himself at the cross and paid for every one of them. The penalty we deserved was poured out on him. Paul explains, "God made him who had no sin to be sin for us, so that in him we might become the righteousness of God" (2 Corinthians 5:21). That's the greatest swap in all of history: on the cross, Christ took our sins, and he gave us his right standing before God.

Does Christ provide happiness for the existentialist? Yes, but not what he expects. Through a transfusion of the blood of Jesus, he can become utterly realistic about life. He no longer has to fear difficulties because now he's assured God is with him through them all. The process of spiritual growth for the existentialist is the deepening realization that he can trust God's goodness and greatness to lead him and use him to accomplish God's purposes. Gradually, Christ's prayer in the garden becomes his own: "Not my will, Father, but yours."

Does Christ offer security for the moralist? Certainly, but Jesus doesn't give him even more rules to follow. When moralists repent, those who formerly kept rules to prove their value now find the courage to look inside and realize they can never do enough to earn God's acceptance. His forgiveness and love are given freely. They finally understand that they can't check off enough boxes of obedience to twist his arm and gain leverage with him. When they realize that life is all grace, not proving their value by their efforts, they can relax. They begin loving people they had condemned, they are humble instead of boasting in their superior deeds and values, and they experience the sheer thrill of being forgiven! They learn that rules have their place, but it's not *first* place. God gave laws to us as a tutor (Galatians 3:24) to show us how far we fall short of God's standard of perfection so that we long to be forgiven. And he gives believers directives so we can channel our passion to please the One who bought us (Titus

2:11-14). Obedience isn't a *means* of grace, but a *result* of grace in our lives.

When existentialists and moralists experience the blood of Jesus and are transformed, they gain a new motivation and power that transforms relationships. Their former superiority, apathy, and resentment are overwhelmed by the love of God, and they express their love in countless ways. The deeper we let Christ's forgiveness sink into us, the more we'll forgive, love, and accept those around us—even our enemies. Paul wrote to the Ephesians, "Get rid of all bitterness, rage and anger, brawling and slander, along with every form of malice. Be kind and compassionate to one another, forgiving each other, just as in Christ God forgave you" (Ephesians 4:31-32). To whom will we show kindness and compassion? The same ones we've been bitter toward before. Christ's love and forgiveness changes us, and through us, it changes our relationships.

Transformation

Unless we have a disease, the red cells in our bodies function automatically to carry oxygen and nutrition to our cells and eliminate poisonous waste. In spiritual life, however, the transfer doesn't happen quite as naturally. Throughout the Bible, the writers encourage us to think, consider, ponder, and remember. Paul wrote to the Christians in Rome: "Therefore, I urge you, brothers, in view of God's mercy, to offer your bodies as living sacrifices, holy and pleasing to God—this is your spiritual act of worship. Do not conform any longer to the pattern of this world, but be transformed by the renewing of your mind. Then you will be able to test and approve what God's will is—his good, pleasing and perfect will" (Romans 12:1-2). For eleven chapters, he had described the importance of the blood of Jesus to change our lives, and now, in light of all they had learned in those chapters, he urges them to renew their minds so they can make good choices to honor God. When we consider the blood of Jesus, we won't be passive. The depth of his love that drove him to give his life for us either astonishes us, or we reject him and walk away. The message of his shed blood cuts deep into our hearts, exposing our selfishness and arrogance, and it reminds us that we were doomed to eternal death without his payment on the cross. We simply can't be apathetic about the pivotal point in all of history and in each of our lives.

As we let our minds think about the cross, our hearts feast on his love. Gradually, we want to know him and please him even more. The worldly things that used to mean so much to us now fade in importance. And when the Holy Spirit taps us on the shoulder to show us an attitude, word, or action that makes him sad, we don't make excuses. We confess our sin and apply the forgiveness we've already received to that sin. In his first letter, John wrote, "If we claim to be without sin, we deceive ourselves and the truth is not in us. If we confess our sins, he is faithful and just and will forgive us our sins and purify us from all unrighteousness" (1 John 1:8-9). Confession means "to agree with." When we confess our sins, we agree that we've done or said something wrong, that Christ's blood already has forgiven us, and that we want to choose a new habit that honors God. Confession doesn't make us forgiven—Christ has already accomplished that feat—but it makes his forgiveness real in our present experience.

When we have the courage to be honest with God about our sins—even those we've never admitted to anyone before—an amazing thing happens. The Spirit of God gives us a transfusion of Christ's love and forgiveness, and he changes our hearts, our motives, our desires, and our direction in life. As he described the way the gospel changes our hearts, Paul almost drifted into ecstasy. He wrote to the Corinthians, "Now the Lord is the Spirit, and where the Spirit of the Lord is, there is freedom. And we, who with unveiled faces all reflect the Lord's glory, are being transformed into his likeness with ever-increasing glory, which comes from the Lord, who is the Spirit" (2 Corinthians 3:17-18). We can't reflect the Lord's glory if we hide in shame because we're unwilling to take our sins to Christ. But when we respond to his great love and pour out our hearts to him, he meets us where we are, forgives and accepts us, and changes our lives. We never have to wear a mask when we go to God. He already knows everything about us—even the very worst things we've tried to hide our whole lives—and he loves us dearly.

The cycle of spiritual life cleanses out the garbage of resentment and superiority and fills us with a beautiful love for others. Richard is a prominent attorney who, by his own admission, had been an incorrigibly selfish alcoholic for many years. A few years ago, he hit rock bottom and turned his life over to Christ. He had a lot to learn in his new life. He explained, "Even though I was a drunk, I always looked down on people who weren't as smart, good-looking, or successful as I was. Yeah, I know—it was the height of hypocrisy."

For Richard, being judgmental was a way of life, and one that didn't evaporate when he became a Christian. To change, he had to develop a new pattern of thinking and acting. When harsh, superior, judgmental thoughts came into his mind, he learned to look squarely at the person and say to himself, "That's someone Jesus died for." Recently, he explained that he had always made fun of a particular group of people. In fact, he had avoided them at all costs. He told me, "But I realized it's sin to avoid people Jesus loves. I decided to go out of my way to make eye contact and speak to each of these people. It's made all the difference in the world. They really appreciate the attention I give them, and I've begun to see them as real people instead of cardboard cutouts. The love of God does amazing things."

On the cellular, molecular, and atomic levels in our bodies, change happens continuously at an amazing pace as particles are created and discarded, oxygen fuels the motors of the cells, and harmful waste is carried off to be eliminated. In the spiritual world, God has given us a wealth of nourishment in his love and power, and his forgiveness cancels out the most horrible, destructive toxins in our lives. Like the continuous flow of red cells in our blood vessels, God's love, forgiveness, and strength never stop flowing into us. But unlike the circulatory system, we need to recognize God's presence to fully experience the wonder of his love. God wants us to be actively involved in the transformation process. If we fail to stimulate the exchange of spiritual nourishment and elimination, we become spiritually anemic—weak, exhausted, and with potential heart disease. But when we learn to think deeply and accurately about the incredible love, power, and forgiveness in the blood of Christ, we let his grace sink deep into every part of our spiritual lives—and he changes us from the inside out.

Think about it...

1. How do red cells nourish our bodies? How do they eliminate waste?

2. Read 1 John 1:7-9. How does the blood of Christ spiritually perform these same functions?

3. How would you define and describe spiritual anemia?

4. What are some negative evidences of romantic existentialism in spiritual life? What are some evidences of rule-keeping moralism? Is either of these a struggle for you? If so, explain your answer.

5. When was a time in your life when you felt nourished by the love and power of Christ's sacrifice? How did it affect you at that point?

6. Why is brutal honesty about sin a prerequisite to experience Christ's forgiveness?

7. How do Christ's love, forgiveness, and power transform our lives?

White Cells: Protection

" In some ways, our white blood cells are better Christians

than we are. These cells have one mission, one purpose—

to give their lives in defense of ours. Why do we doubt

[Christ's] vigilance when he so faithfully performs it on the

microscopic level every day of our lives? The evidence

is overwhelming—he sees, he cares, and he defends."

—Richard Swenson, M. D.

White blood cells are the sentries and soldiers in our bodies. They are always on the lookout for danger, and they actively fight for us every second of our lives. These cells, also called *leuco-cytes*, consist of various classes of specialized cells, each with specific functions essential to life and health. White cells live not only in the bloodstream, but also throughout our bodies. What are they searching for and fighting against so valiantly? Our bodies contain a myriad of microorganisms: bacteria, viruses, and fungi. In addition, we also have abnormal particles, such as dust, carbon, allergens, and by-products from cellular biochemical reactions and environmental toxins floating around in our bodies. Many of the bacteria in our bodies are essential to life, such as the ones in our guts that aid digestion. Some microbes, like flu viruses, are noxious and make us sick, and others, such as Ebola and other virulent versions, can prove to be fatal.

Surveillance and Defense

White cells don't just stand by and watch these microbes float past them. They sacrifice themselves every moment of our lives to kill any threat. In the movie *Outbreak*, the military and Centers for Disease Control gave a briefing about the potential spread of the deadly microbe. In a few hours, it would spread to neighboring states; in a few days, to the whole country; and in less than a week, across the globe. This fiction isn't far from reality. Microbes may live only a few minutes, but they multiply at an astronomical rate. They are the most numerous and prolific form of life on earth. A study by Dr. Darold Treffort reports that if these microbes were "allowed to go unchecked for only thirty-six hours, they would reproduce in numbers that could cover the entire planet to a thickness of over a foot."[14]

Our skin and mucus membranes in our noses, mouths, and digestive tracts are our first line of defense against attacks. When these are breached, white cells from our blood and other tissues race to the scene in seconds to engage in mortal combat. The sentries and soldiers in our bodies number about fifty billion, but one hundred times this number are waiting in our bone marrow to be called up for duty. Specialized white cells focus on particular intruders: *neutrophils* combat bacteria, *T and B cell lymphocytes* fight viruses, and both kinds of white cells war against fungi.

---

14 Darold A. Treffort, M. D., *Extraordinary People: Understanding Savant Syndrome,* (New York: Ballentine Books, 1989), pp. 1, 2, 59.

In a microscopic scene that looks more like *Star Wars* than the world we see each day, white cells envelop the intruders in a process called *phagocytosis*, and then, with deadly force, a lysosome enzyme kills it. In this process, billions of molecular receptors identify the intruder, create antibodies, attach to the microbes, and execute them.

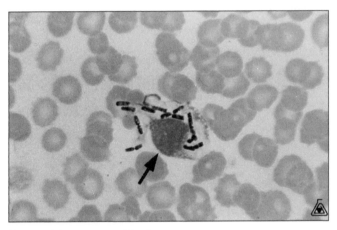

Figure 6. Monocyte engulfing bacteria.

We may become annoyed when we get a fever, swollen lymph nodes, a sore throat, or pus around an infection, but all of these are signs that billions of white blood cells have come to our rescue to fight and die for us. Usually, we're aware of this fight only when we get sick, and even then, we assume our bodies have let us down. The truth is that they are working marvelously well when we have those symptoms, but they are working almost as hard every second of our lives as they perform "search and destroy" missions to protect us. If our white cells stopped their constant surveillance and protection, we'd die within ten minutes.

Two specialized white cells are B cells and T cells. B cells patrol the bloodstream and lymph system looking for enemy combatants, and when they find them, they produce antibodies to fight and kill them.

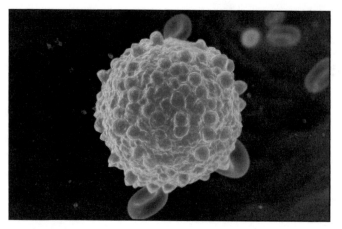

Figure 7. B cell.

T cells have a long memory, recognizing destructive microbes to-day that may not enter the person's body for decades. Over the course of a long life, the immune system develops an extensive library of sub-stances and microbes that are catalogued as "a threat" or "not a threat." Long after the previous infection, T cells instantly recognize any new exposure to the pathogen and attack it (see Figure 8).

When someone coughs next to you on the bus, at work, or in church, you inhale some of the person's microbes suspended in the air. If any of the microbes get past the mucous membrane in your nose or throat, the T cells may recognize that it's a microbe that made you sick in the past. In an instant, the T cells give instructions to the B cells to produce antibodies to attack and kill it. While scientists studied AIDS and similar diseases and disorders, they discovered that

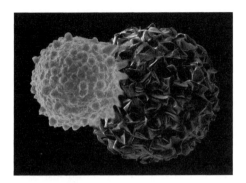

Figure 8. T cell.

the body has the ability to regulate the production of various types of cells. It even has the capacity to mutate fully developed, functioning B cells into T cells.

I talk to worried mothers who are very concerned that their little children are "getting too many colds and ear infections." I tell them not to fret. Each illness in infancy is producing a stockpile of effective T cells that will prevent more serious infections as the child grows up. In fact, some of the worst sicknesses in adults can be the result of the person being too closely protected as a child. I'm not advocating that parents not treat the symptoms. Certainly, that's appropriate, but don't be too worried about normal childhood sicknesses. See each one as another deposit in the T cell bank for the future.

Some concerned parents today are opponents of child immunizations that are designed to boost the immune system. Their resistance, I believe, is misguided. They should travel to Africa and other undeveloped parts of the world to see the utter devastation caused by easily preventable serious childhood diseases, such as measles and diphtheria. My message to these parents is simple: don't be foolish; immunize your children.

Most people think of cancer only in its advanced state when it threatens health and life, but the body produces abnormal cells all the time. White cells routinely destroy them, and it's only when abnormal cells multiply too rapidly or the white cells fail to kill enough of them (which is more likely as we age) that the abnormal cells become a serious threat. For new treatments and prevention, doctors are trying to identify the genes that enable white cells to effectively eliminate abnormal cells so they don't multiply into cancer. Recent advances in immunotherapy promise new vaccines that can be produced from a patient's own cancer cells. These vaccines will specifically target and destroy cancerous cells and preserve normal cells, greatly reducing the side effects and morbidity of chemotherapy.

People with diabetes often lose fingers, toes, feet, and legs to amputation because high levels of glucose damage their blood vessels, a condition which limits the supply of blood to their extremities. The lack of blood supply decreases oxygen delivery and the tissue becomes necrotic (dead). When they get an infection, their bodies aren't able to transport enough white cells to that part of their bodies, and the infection becomes much more severe, often gangrenous. When the infection kills too much healthy tissue, amputation may become the only option.

In rare cases, white cells get it wrong. Like soldiers who are the victims of "friendly fire," the immune system in some people attacks healthy cells, leading to debilitating illnesses and sometimes death. When the body identifies healthy cells as pathogens, it unleashes all the destructive power of the white cells against itself. Rheumatoid arthritis and multiple sclerosis are two of the most common forms of autoimmune disease, but more than eighty exist. Autoimmune diseases are among the ten leading causes of death among women in all age groups up to 65 years.[15]

---

15 Noel R. Rose and Ian R. MacKay, *The Autoimmune Diseases,* Fourth Edition.

We are seldom aware of the protection provided for us by our white blood cells. Every moment, they win the Congressional Medal of Honor for giving their lives so that we can live. They are a powerful metaphor of God's protection of us.

Our Refuge and Strength

We don't live in the Garden God intended us to enjoy. Because of sin, our world is fallen, and we're part of that fallen cosmos. When we suffer, some of us blame God for not making our lives as smooth as silk, but he never promised that he'd eliminate the natural consequences of living in a fallen world or the results of our poor choices. In our disappointment, we may see God as distant, angry, or condemning. However, as we understand the message of the gospel and the blood sacrificed by Jesus on the cross, we'll realize that God is our defender and father, a "very present help in time of trouble."

One of the key concepts in the Bible is that our sins deserve the wrath of God, but because of Christ's payment on the cross, all the wrath of God was poured out on him there. Now, with our sins completely forgiven, God directs all of his love and compassion toward us. At one point, the people of God accused God of forgetting about them. He replied with tender correction:

> *"Can a mother forget the baby at her breast*
> *and have no compassion on the child she has borne?*
> *Though she may forget,*
> *I will not forget you!*
> *See, I have engraved you on the palms of my hands"*
> *(Isaiah 49:15-16).*

Like the constant vigilance of our white cells, God's love and care for us never ceases, even when we don't realize it's there. In a beautiful psalm of God's constant care, the ancient writer tells us:

"He who dwells in the shelter of the Most High
will rest in the shadow of the Almighty.
I will say of the LORD, 'He is my refuge and my fortress,
my God, in whom I trust.'
Surely he will save you from the fowler's snare
and from the deadly pestilence" (Psalm 91:1-3).

Notice the words he uses to describe God's nature: shelter, shadow, refuge, and fortress. We can turn to him when we face difficulties, even a physical, spiritual, or relational "deadly pestilence." The battles we fight in our spiritual lives are, like the pathogens our white cells war against, both internal and external. Inside us, we fight against indwelling sin, our natural "bent" to go our own way, reject God, and live for our own pleasures. External attacks come from the enemy of our souls, Satan and his dark angels. Let's look at both types.

Attacks from inside

The most significant pathogenic threat to people isn't what comes to them from the outside; it's the attacks they experience from the microbes that live inside them. In the spiritual world, the internal pathogens are our sinful desires. Paul explained to the believers in Galatia that they could expect a fierce and constant battle with their sinful natures. He wrote, "So I say, live by the Spirit, and you will not gratify the desires of the sinful nature. For the sinful nature desires what is contrary to the Spirit, and the Spirit what is contrary to the sinful nature. They are in conflict with each other, so that you do not do what you want" (Galatians 5:16-17). Are you fighting against desires to be selfish, arrogant, or cowardly? Welcome to the club. That's a normal part of life. It's only a problem if we fail to fight well. Paul continued to explain that a good grasp of the death of Christ gives us insight, power, and courage to fight well. He wrote, "Those who belong to Christ Jesus have crucified the sinful nature with its passions and desires. Since we live by the Spirit, let us keep in step with the Spirit" (verses 24-25). The blood of Jesus gives us a new identity as children of the King, a new direction to honor him, and a new power to enable us to overcome selfish passions so that we love God with all our hearts and love others as we love ourselves—but it's always a fight.

Attacks from the outside

Our struggle, however, isn't just with internal spiritual microbes. We fight against a vicious and ancient external enemy. At the end of his enlightening letter to the Ephesian Christians, Paul told them bluntly, "Finally, be strong in the Lord and in his mighty power. Put on the full armor of God so that you can take your stand against the devil's schemes. For our struggle is not against flesh and blood, but against the rulers, against the authorities, against the powers of this dark world and against the spiritual forces of evil in the heavenly realms" (Ephesians 6:10-12). Satan's schemes to throw us off track are deception, temptation, and accusation.

• *Deception*

Paul reminded us that Satan "disguises himself as an angel of light." Our enemy casts doubt on the faithfulness of God, the power of the cross, the depth of God's love, and the Lord's purpose for our lives. When we're not paying attention, he whispers in our ears the same question he asked Eve, "Has God really said that? Does he really care? You can't trust him with your deepest desires, can you?" And when he whispers to us, he uses our own voice, so it sounds completely reasonable. Virtually all the cults began when a doctrine of the church became twisted—even just slightly—into an untruth.

It's not just cults that are sources of deception. In one of Jesus' most famous parables, the one about the four soils, he explained, "The one who received the seed that fell among the thorns is the man who hears the word, but the worries of this life and the deceitfulness of wealth choke it, making it unfruitful" (Matthew 13:22). Our worries are an indication that we think we know more than God about how he should run the universe and how he should treat us. We worry about things we can control, but even more, about things we can't control. One of our chief worries is money. We compulsively compare our lives with others to see if we have enough possessions, positions, and popularity so we can feel superior (or at least, not inferior). But the pursuit of riches steals our hearts away from God, slowly poisoning our hearts with misplaced affections. Paul reminded Timothy that the love of money, not money itself, is the root of all evil (1 Timothy 6:10).

- *Temptation*

Another spiritual pathogen Satan wants to use to infect our hearts is temptation. The thought or momentary desire for sex or power or pleasure is entirely normal for a living, breathing human being, just as it's normal for microbes to exist for a short time in the body before being identified and killed by white blood cells. But like the white cells, we have to identify the temptation quickly, surround it with truth, and eradicate it from our hearts. If we let it multiply, it will consume us and destroy us. James told us, "When tempted, no one should say, 'God is tempting me.' For God cannot be tempted by evil, nor does he tempt anyone; but each one is tempted when, by his own evil desire, he is dragged away and enticed. Then, after desire has conceived, it gives birth to sin; and sin, when it is full-grown, gives birth to death" (James 1:13-15). That's pretty close to a description of a virus that takes hold in the body, overwhelms the defenses, and kills the patient.

Each of us experiences a particular pattern of temptation. Some feel intense longing for corporate promotion, some long for approval and praise, and many can't stop thinking about sex. Temptation, however, isn't just about the "big sins." We're tempted to gossip because it makes us feel superior to the person we're talking about, we're tempted to seek revenge instead of forgiving because getting back at people is so intoxicating, and when we experience hardships, we're tempted to doubt God's goodness and wisdom, so we wallow in self-pity. As soon as we realize we're letting our minds dwell on the "what ifs" and "what abouts," we need to arrest those thoughts and replace them with powerful truths about God's love, grace, sacrifice, and purpose for us. As long as we're in this world, we won't escape the reality of temptation. However, just as our white cells fight for us until the day we die, we can fight well and fight hard to overcome temptation one at a time. Facing the tests of temptation makes us stronger and able to combat the evil desires even better the next time.

- *Accusation*

Another ploy of the evil one is to accuse us of being unworthy, unfit, and unlovable. Again, the voice sounds like our own, so we don't even realize it's an attack from the enemy. We call ourselves horrible names, and though we try to put on a smile when we're with others, we secretly fear what they think of us. In our insecurity, we wear masks to cover up our self-doubts while we project to others that we're the kings and queens of the world. We don't win the battle against accusations by trying to prove ourselves, but with humility and honesty. When we hear a voice that says, "You're scum," we can reply, "Yes, but Jesus Christ loves me enough to die for me, so I'm something to him." When we hear the accusation, "You'll never amount to anything," we respond, "I'm God's workmanship, created in Christ Jesus for good works." Our response to every accusation is to go back to the cross, to remember that the blood of Jesus pays for all our sins, qualifies us to be God's beloved children, and gives us a new, powerful sense of purpose.

Developing spiritual T cells

Each time we battle successfully with indwelling sin or external attacks by Satan, we develop the spiritual equivalent of T cells in our hearts. The next time we're tempted, deceived, or accused, we remember, we instantly realize, "I've been here before. Even if I didn't handle it very well last time, at least I learned some lessons, and I can handle it better this time." Our use of Scripture, prayer, and the power of the Spirit are unleashed like B cell antibodies to attack the specific problem. We study the Bible to find out more about God's nature, the depth of his forgiveness, and his will for us in every situation, and we trust his Spirit to give us the power and love we need to fulfill his will. As we've seen, throughout the Bible, God instructs us to remember. In the *shema*, the most significant direction to the children of Israel, a statement to be repeated throughout their lives and throughout history, Moses tells the people to memorize, rehearse, and repeat this statement of faith:

"Hear, O Israel: The LORD our God, the LORD is one. Love the LORD your God with all your heart and with all your soul and with all your strength. These commandments that I give

you today are to be upon your hearts. Impress them on your children. Talk about them when you sit at home and when you walk along the road, when you lie down and when you get up. Tie them as symbols on your hands and bind them on your foreheads. Write them on the doorframes of your houses and on your gates" (Deuteronomy 6:4-9).

After Moses died, God appointed Joshua to lead the people to the Promised Land. The people stood on the banks of the Jordan River, and when the priests put their feet in the water, the river dried up so the people could cross on dry ground. The priests carried the ark into the middle of the riverbed and stood as the people of God walked by. God dried the Red Sea for Moses, and now he dried the Jordan River for Joshua. After the last person had crossed, God told Joshua to build a memorial: "Choose twelve men from among the people, one from each tribe, and tell them to take up twelve stones from the middle of the Jordan from right where the priests stood and to carry them over with you and put them down at the place where you stay tonight" (Joshua 4:2-3).

A man from each tribe put a stone on a pile at the campsite. That night, Joshua told the people, "In the future when your descendants ask their fathers, 'What do these stones mean?' tell them, 'Israel crossed the Jordan on dry ground.' For the LORD your God dried up the Jordan before you until you had crossed over. The LORD your God did to the Jordan just what he had done to the Red Sea when he dried it up before us until we had crossed over. He did this so that all the peoples of the earth might know that the hand of the LORD is powerful and so that you might always fear the LORD your God" (Joshua 4:21-24). Every spiritual victory is like putting a stone on our heart's memorial to God's grace, power, and faithfulness. And as the pile of stones gets higher and wider, our memories—and our defenses against future attacks—become stronger.

To strengthen our spiritual immune systems, God exposes us to all kinds of struggles—not to crush us, but to strengthen us (see James 1:2-4). Seasons of struggle, pruning, drought, and spiritually fallow ground are important parts of God's will and his ways in our lives. We naturally try to avoid pain at all costs, but in pushing it away, we miss God's purpose for it. In his seminal work, *Knowing God*, professor J. I. Packer observed that God has a higher purpose than helping us avoid pain. He wrote,

> *"This is what all the work of grace aims at—an even deeper knowledge of God, and an ever closer fellowship with Him. Grace is God drawing us sinners closer and closer to Him. How does God in grace prosecute this purpose? Not by shielding us from assault by the world, the flesh, and the devil, nor by protecting us from burdensome and frustrating circumstances, nor yet by shielding us from troubles created by our own temperament and psychology; but rather by exposing us to all these things, so as to overwhelm us with a sense of our own inadequacy, and to drive us to cling to Him more closely. This is the ultimate reason, from our standpoint, why God fills our lives with troubles and perplexities of one sort or another—it is to ensure that we shall learn to hold Him fast."[16]*

Pathogens can cause us to die, or they can trigger a process of creating T cells that protect us for years to come. In the same way, the

---

16 J. I. Packer, *Knowing God,* (Intervarsity Press, Downer's Grove, Ill., 1973), p. 227.

heartaches we face can destroy us, or we can trust God to use them to make us stronger.

Friendship as T cells and B cells

To change the metaphor a bit, I believe that close relationships in the body of Christ serve as effective T cells to protect each person from harm. When we "speak the truth in love," we offer words of affirmation and correction, "according to the need of the moment." A true friend finds the courage to step into our lives to say the hard things that need to be said. When we're going off track, we desperately need someone to care enough to be God's voice of loving rebuke. Some people are like B cells that react to a particular threat in our lives to help us, but others remain like T cells for many years, sharing wisdom and protecting us from recurring difficulties we face over the years.

Paul wrote the Galatians, "Carry each other's burdens, and in this way you will fulfill the law of Christ" (Galatians 6:2). White cells are born to "carry one another's burdens" and give their lives for the good of others. When we love one another the way Christ loves us, we'll be willing to step into people's lives to protect them from the destructive pathogens of personal sin and the attacks of the enemy.

Leaders are often isolated from close relationships because they are perceived as powerful and unapproachable. I believe that leaders must find someone to love them enough to speak the truth to them—especially if they don't want to hear it. In ancient times, a powerful general in the Roman army often led his forces to glorious victories. When he rode through the streets to the cheers of the adoring throngs, he realized he had to find someone to keep him from becoming arrogant. He hired a man to whisper into his ear three times an hour, "Remember, you are just a man."

God has given me some wonderful people during my life to affirm and redirect me. At times, they saw gifts and abilities in me that I didn't even notice, and their encouragement propelled me to a new level of effectiveness as a husband, father, doctor, and pastor. At other times, they spoke hard words to me, words of warning that I needed to hear. And sometimes, they imparted life to me. When I was ten years old, my mother died and my world came crashing down. I was devastated. A man in our neighborhood gave me a job delivering papers. At a time when my family was fractured, this man believed in me and showed confidence in me.

For years after my mother died, I was furious. She meant the world to me, but after being sick only a day, she was gone. The experience of loss at that young age, however, gave me a tender heart toward others who are hurting. Since that tragic day when I was a child, I've been well aware that life is terribly fragile, and I've had a sense of urgency to make a difference while I'm alive. This painful experience played a major role in me becoming a doctor and a pastor. I would never have chosen that hard school of learning, but God used it to shape my life in powerful ways. Still, through all the pain of those years and the joys of serving as a physician and a pastor, I've needed the honesty and love of a few people to make me the person God wants me to be. Who has God sent to be spiritual T and B cells in your life?

Unseen Protection

As a physician, I have a front row seat on the majesty of God's creation. Every day, I see intricacies and wonders of the human body that most people never notice. If we were aware of the fight being waged in our bodies at this very moment, we'd be amazed at the goodness of God to create billions of white blood cells to stand guard over every tissue and sacrifice their lives to protect us from harm. In the spiritual world, I'm convinced that the same thing is happening right now. God continually protects his children from internal and external attacks. A few of them surface and come into view from time to time, but most of them remain hidden. At every moment of every day, we can be sure that God is always at work as our shelter, defender, and refuge.

Throughout history, God has given a glimpse of the unseen world from time to time. In the centuries after King David, the nation of Israel was conquered by several nations, including the Babylonians, the Persians, and the Assyrians. The prophet Elisha spoke out boldly for God, no matter what the consequences might be. When the Arameans threatened to attack, he warned the king of Israel to be prepared. The king of Aram was furious, and he sent a strong army and many chariots against the lone prophet of God. The next morning, Elisha's servant went out early and saw the vast army surrounding them. He panicked, "Oh, my lord, what shall we do?" (2 Kings 6:15)

"Don't be afraid," the prophet answered. "Those who are with us are more than those who are with them." Elisha prayed, "O LORD, open his eyes so he may see." The historian tells us, "Then the LORD opened the servant's eyes, and he looked and saw the hills full of horses and chariots of fire all around Elisha" (2 Kings 6:15-17).

When I look through a microscope or see the therapeutic effects of an antibiotic on an infection, my eyes are opened to see the power of God at work on the cellular level. With this assurance, I can trust that God is powerfully at work in my life and in the lives of those I love even when I can't see it with my eyes. I have no idea how much God protects us from each day, but I'm sure it's a lot! On this side of heaven, we'll never know all the ways God "leads us not into temptation" and "delivers us from evil," but understanding the amazing warrior qualities of white blood cells gives me a clue.

Are you ever tempted to doubt God's constant care? Do you wonder if he's paying attention at all? If you have these doubts, you're in good company. The people of Israel suffered through domination at the hands of cruel nations. After a while, they felt sorry for themselves. They complained, "My way is hidden from the LORD; my cause is disregarded by my God."

Like a wise, patient, and persistent teacher, the prophet Isaiah reminded them of God's continual care. First, he admonished them:

"Do you not know?

> *Have you not heard?*

> *The LORD is the everlasting God,*

> *the Creator of the ends of the earth.*

He will not grow tired or weary,

> *and his understanding no one can fathom."*

He then tells them again of God's love and faithfulness:

"He gives strength to the weary

> *and increases the power of the weak.*

Even youths grow tired and weary,

> *and young men stumble and fall;*

but those who hope in the LORD

> *will renew their strength.*

> *They will soar on wings like eagles;*

> *they will run and not grow weary,*

> *they will walk and not be faint" (Isaiah 40:27-31).*

When we feel attacked, Isaiah reminds us to focus our hearts on the goodness, love, and power of God. Then we can have hope. The death of Christ is proof to us that God's love never falters. After describing the glory of the cross to the people in Rome, Paul almost shouts, "If God is for us, who can be against us? He who did not spare his own Son, but gave him up for us all—how will he not also, along with him, graciously give us all things?" (Romans 8:31-32) In other words, if God has given us the very most he could possibly give, we can surely trust him to give us everything else we truly need.

In this life, we won't escape attacks by microbes, sinful desires, and Satan's schemes, but we can have strong hope that God never gets tired of loving us, protecting us, and giving us all we need to trust him for today. The sacrifice of Jesus is his sovereign covenant, "the new covenant in my blood," to assure us that he knows, he cares, and he is with us whether our hearts soar like eagles, we run the race with endurance, or we can only put one foot in front of the other as we walk with him through hard times.

One of the most beautiful and powerful hymns about the blood of Jesus is "When I Survey the Wondrous Cross," penned by Isaac Watts. Let the message sink deep into your soul:

"When I survey the wondrous cross
on which the Prince of Glory died;
my richest gain I count but loss,
and pour contempt on all my pride.

Forbid it, Lord, that I should boast,
save in the death of Christ, my God;
all the vain things that charm me most,
I sacrifice them to his blood.

See, from his head, his hands, his feet,
sorrow and love flow mingled down.
Did e'er such love and sorrow meet,
or thorns compose so rich a crown.

Were the whole realm of nature mine,
that were an offering far too small;
love so amazing, so divine,
demands my soul, my life, my all." [17]

Think about it...

1. Does it scare you or excite you that you have so many microbes in your body right now? Explain your answer.

---

17   "When I Survey the Wondrous Cross," lyrics by Isaac Watts, music by Lowell Mason.

2. Why is it important that T cells have long memories of past infections?

3. What does the fight against the internal pathogen of indwelling sin look like in your life today? What do you need to do to fight and win?

4. What do you need to fight deception, temptation, and accusation more effectively?

5. In what way does God's grace use our struggles to make us stronger? How is that like T cells?

6. What do you need to remember about God when you are tempted to complain?

Platelets: Healing the Hurts

" God whispers to us in our pleasures, speaks in our con-

sciences, but shouts in our pain: it is His megaphone to

rouse a deaf world."

—C. S. Lewis

When we experience any kind of injury, our platelets are the EMS truck that rushes to the scene. Whether the injury is internal where we can't see it, or external, breaking the skin, the delicate capillaries are ruptured. Blood loss is a serious threat to our bodies, and platelets are God's first response team whose role is to stop the flow and begin the healing process.

First at the Scene

Platelets are irregularly shaped, sticky, colorless cells that survive only a few days. For that reason, we produce five million new platelets every second. As soon as a wound occurs, platelets and other substances rush immediately to the scene to block the flow of blood. Calcium, vitamin K, and a protein called *fibrinogen* are essential to the formation of a clot. The clot, though, isn't a simple plug. A sequence of at least twelve stages is involved in a complex biochemical reaction to form the initial clot and transform it into permanent healing. Platelets are produced in the bone marrow—the same as the red cells and most of the white blood cells—from very large bone marrow cells called *megakaryocytes*, which fragment and release thousands of platelets.

Platelets are the smallest and lightest of the types of blood cells. Like tiny debris in a fast-flowing stream, they are pushed from the center of flowing blood to the wall of the blood vessel, which is lined by cells called *endothelium*. The endothelium has a surface similar to Teflon that prevents anything from sticking to it. When an injury occurs, the endothelial layer ruptures, and the fibers that surround a blood vessel are exposed to the flowing blood. That's the signal for platelets to spring into action. The fibers surrounding the vessel wall attract platelets and stimulate the creation of tiny threads, called *fibrin*, which begin the process of clotting to stop the flow of blood (see Figure 9).

For example, when a child falls and scrapes her knee, blood vessels in the skin constrict, and fibrinogen in the platelets immediately begin to form tiny threads. These thread weave together to form a mesh to hold the blood and keep it from flowing out of the body. In a few minutes, blood stops oozing from the scrape. As the threads harden in the next couple of hours, they form a clot. On the surface of the body, this clot is an *eschar*, more commonly called a scab. Over time, the healing process under the scab closes the wound and restores the tissues. If the child picks the scab off and reopens the

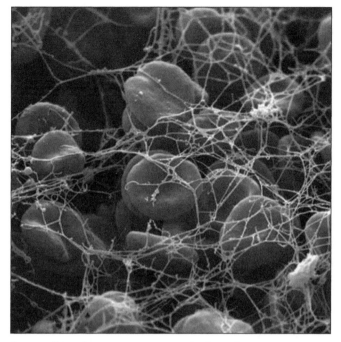

Figure 9. Fibrin forming a web to stop the flow of blood.

wound, the entire process begins again. If she leaves it alone, the broken vessels and skin will heal completely in a matter of days.

We can easily identify scabs on the skin as evidence of the work of platelets, and in internal injuries, they work much the same way to stop the flow of blood. When blood vessels are ruptured without breaking the skin, platelets rush to the scene to stop the flow. Near the surface of the skin, we notice these clots as bruises, but internal organs can also experience bruising we never see. Some internal clots can be dangerous if they block the flow of blood to a vital area or break off and flow into the bloodstream to the heart, lungs, or brain. A clot that lodges in an artery in the brain causes a stroke, cutting off or severely reducing the flow of blood and life-sustaining oxygen to that part of the brain, leading to temporary or permanent brain damage, paralysis, or death.

Contrary to popular belief, *hemophilia* isn't the absence of the platelets' ability to form a clot, but the inability to complete the long sequence of clot producing steps—actually, the faulty function of a critical coagulation Factor—from surface factors or any of the Factors from I to XI. When hemophiliacs get a wound, their bodies immediately form the initial clot at the site of the wound, but the first stage of clotting only lasts about four hours. When a subsequent stage fails to perform, the wound opens and the person begins bleeding again. This demonstrates to us the critical need for *each component* of the body of Christ to function properly to ensure health and wholeness of everyone (see Ephesians 4:16).

Idiopathic thrombocytopenic purpura (ITP) is a condition in which the platelet count is lower than normal because the immune system attacks and destroys healthy platelets. The normal platelet count is between 150,000–400,000 per cubic millimeter of blood. ITP patients have counts as low or lower than 20,000. The most visible symptoms of this disease are purple bruises on the skin or mucous membranes in the mouth as small vessels rupture and aren't repaired. The bleeding may appear as a rash. The most severe bleeding, however, is intracranial, which may result from a blow to the head. For these patients, any cut, even a simple nosebleed, can prove to be dangerous because their bodies can't stop the bleeding. ITP can be caused by a reaction to some drugs, infections, leukemia, or when the body has exhausted its platelet supply. The body may mistake platelets for a virus, so it produces antibodies to attack and kill the platelets. People with ITP may produce more platelets than the rest of us, but their white cells mistakenly kill them in huge quantities.

The blood's capacity to utilize platelets and clotting factors is the first step in healing. Many sincere believers fail to appreciate the full range of the ways God heals. Some never think about the spiritual dimension of physical healing, and a few misguided people insist that modern medicine is an adversary of God's intentions. There are, I believe, four ways God may choose to heal broken bodies:

1. By far, the most common means of healing is the one we've examined in this chapter: God has beautifully orchestrated human blood to stop internal and external bleeding, fight microbes, and heal hurts—many of which we're not even aware.

2. In a display of common grace, God has given the medical profession incredible advances in our understanding of the body, of the nature of diseases, and recently, into the mysteries of DNA. He often uses doctors to accomplish his will to heal our hurts.

3. Does God still perform genuine miracles of supernatural healing? Yes, of course he does. Though I'm a physician, I've often seen God bring healing when the person's body and medical science have proven inadequate. Sometimes, God chooses to heal like he did when Jesus cleansed lepers, gave sight to the blind, and made sick people well, but sometimes God chooses not to heal. There's nothing wrong in asking God for a miracle as long as we don't demand a particular response. It may take more faith to accept a no than a yes.

4. Even those Jesus healed eventually died. There is coming a day, though, when there will be no more sickness, pain, and death. Those who endured the most debilitating diseases will have, like all of us who believe in Jesus, "glorified bodies" (1 Corinthians

15:35-58). I'm not sure all that Paul's term means, but I'm certain that our new bodies will be like the one Jesus had when he appeared to the disciples after the resurrection.

Unlike the secret work of red and white cells, we have the privilege of seeing the healing effects of platelets every time we have any kind of injury to our skin or near the surface. If we could use time-lapse photography to see the clot form and healing continue, we'd be amazed at the healing power of platelets in our blood.

Christ's Blood Heals Our Wounds

Many of the emotional and relational wounds we've suffered are self-inflicted, but all of us have been, to some degree, hurt by people we trusted. Some of these hurts are as superficial as the child's scraped knee, but others are as deep, traumatic, and debilitating. We may have suffered sexual abuse, emotional abandonment, or rejection by someone we love. Some of us experienced the sledgehammer blows of violence, and many more felt the continuous sandpaper effects of verbal criticism and condemning looks. A few of us have been hurt so badly, so long that we've become numb to the pain—a dangerous condition that leaves us vulnerable to more wounds. But many others live with such deep, unhealed hurts that we react defensively at even the slightest threat of being hurt again. We are always on the alert, overreacting to any perceived offense.

Christ's offer of healing is open to all of us, but we need to engage him at the point of our deepest hurt. Claiming "it's no big deal" only delays the healing God wants to accomplish in our lives. In the most powerful prophesy about the Messiah who would someday come, Isaiah predicted that healing would come because the Lamb of God would take on our sorrows as well as our sins.

"Surely he took up our infirmities
and carried our sorrows,
yet we considered him stricken by God,
smitten by him, and afflicted.
But he was pierced for our transgressions,
he was crushed for our iniquities;
he punishment that brought us peace was upon him,
and by his wounds we are healed" (Isaiah 53:4-5).

Some may say, "Well, I know someone who got sick and Jesus didn't heal him." The primary healing God accomplishes in our lives is spiritual healing. He mends broken hearts, sets the captive free, and restores sight to the spiritually blind. Someday, he will heal all of his people physically. Modern medicine is a glowing evidence of God's common grace to bring healing to sick and broken bodies, but even if we don't experience physical healing in this life, God promises a New Heaven and New Earth where there will be no disease, no tears, and no evil.

In this life, God doesn't protect us from wounds, but he promises to use our pain in a powerful way to remind us of our desperate need for his grace. And as we trust him with our sorrows, he uses us to show others the depth of his love. In fact, the scars of healing authenticate God's work in us to heal the deep hurts we've experienced. After Christ rose from the tomb that Sunday morning, he appeared to the disciples, but Thomas wasn't in the room that day. When the others told him the incredible news that they had seen Jesus, he grumbled, "Unless I see the nail marks in his hands and put my finger where the nails were, and put my hand into his side, I will not believe it." A week later, the disciples were together again, and Jesus came through the walls to appear to them. He told Thomas, "Put your finger here; see my hands. Reach out your hand and put it into my side. Stop doubting and believe." That was the proof Thomas needed. He fell to his knees and pronounced his renewed faith: "My Lord and my God!" (John 20:25-28)

A friend of mine preached a sermon several years ago called "Show Me Your Wounds." His point was that if we won't show our wounds (or if we mistakenly think we don't have any), people don't know if they can trust us. If we try to hide behind masks, they have reason to doubt if we're sincere about our faith in the Healer. Thomas refused to trust in Jesus until he saw the wounds. We may call him "Doubting Thomas," but I believe he's just like the rest of us. He wanted to see the holes in Jesus' hands and side before he was willing to believe in him.

Many wonderful, mature Christians would say that the richest lessons they've learned in life were in the classroom of suffering. They didn't like the classes, but they treasure the results. Paul certainly endured his share of hardships and rejection. He was beaten, flogged, shipwrecked, stoned, and run out of countless towns as he carried the Good News to the world. At one point, he also suffered some kind of physical illness. He asked God to heal him, but God had other plans. In a letter to the Corinthians, he explained God's purpose for his suffering: "Three times I pleaded with the Lord to take it away from me. But he said to me, 'My grace is sufficient for you, for my power is made perfect in weakness.' Therefore I will boast all the more gladly about my weaknesses, so that Christ's power may rest on me. That is why, for Christ's sake, I delight in weaknesses, in insults, in hardships, in persecutions, in difficulties. For when I am weak, then I am strong" (2 Corinthians 12:8-10). God didn't release Paul from his pain. Instead, God used the pain in his life to authenticate his role as an apostle, deepen his compassion for hurting people, and remind him of Christ's suffering for him. The amazing thing isn't God's intention to use Paul's suffering for good, but Paul's willingness to accept God's will and even delight in it. That's real faith! A friend of mine said, "If you really want to please the Lord by learning from suffering, you don't have to look for it. It already knows your address." Pain is the crucible of growth. We learn far more in the valley than we do on the mountaintop. In his love and his sovereign purpose, God brings a wide range of difficulties into our lives to prune us and stimulate us to grow so we become a little bit more like Jesus.

Wounds will make us bitter, or they'll tenderize our hearts. In the same spirit of hope that God will use our pain to teach us important lessons, author and professor Dan Allender observes,

"If we fail to respond appropriately to the wounds that life and relationships inflict, our pain will be wasted; it will numb us or destroy us. But suffering doesn't have to mangle our hearts and rob us of the joy of life. It can, instead, lead us to life–if we know the path to healing. Healing is not the resolution of our past; it is the use of our past to draw us into deeper relationship with God and his purposes for our lives. We can move from feelings of powerlessness, betrayal, and ambivalence into faith, hope and love."[18]

Forgiveness, Experienced and Expressed

If we allow unhealed hurts to multiply, we experience a churning morass of hurt, anger, fear, and resentment. We're angry with the people who have hurt us, the ones who failed to protect us, the

---

18 Dan Allender, *The Healing Path,* (Water Brook Press, Colorado Springs, Colorado, 1999), pp. 5-6.

people who even look like they might hurt us today, and God because we're sure he should have prevented it. Resentment (and it's first cousin, bitterness) is poisonous, but it gives us two things we desperately want: identity and energy. We think of ourselves as "the one who was wronged," and we delight in people feeling sorry for us or being terrified of our volcanic explosions. And we wake up each day with a fresh shot of adrenaline coursing through our veins. When our minds are at rest, they soon drift to thoughts of revenge. We long to get back at the people who wronged us, but if we're Christians, we become passive-aggressive—we want revenge, but we don't want to get caught!

Author and pastor Frederick Buechner observed, "Of the Seven Deadly Sins, anger is possibly the most fun. To lick your wounds, to smack your lips over grievances long past, to roll over your tongue the prospect of bitter confrontations still to come, to savor to the last toothsome morsel both the pain you are given and the pain you are giving back—in many ways it is a feast fit for a king. The chief drawback is that what you are wolfing down is yourself. The skeleton at the feast is you!"[19] Bitterness is the ultimate spiritual autoimmune disease, producing antibodies to kill even the healthiest parts of us.

For most of us, the problem isn't that we've experienced wounds, but that we've never allowed those wounds to heal. Like ITP attacking life-saving platelets, we sabotage our own healing by stopping the process before it can begin. We cling to our resentment because we believe the identity and energy it provides are more necessary than the freedom, love, and peace we can have if we forgive the offender. We hold tight to the *pathogenic known* because we're afraid of the mysteries of a *healthy unknown*.

---

19 Frederick Buechner, *Wishful Thinking*, (Harper San Francisco, 1993), p. 2.

Learning to give and receive forgiveness is one of the most difficult—and one of the most necessary—aspects of life. Part of being created in the image of God is that he has put a sense of justice in all of us. For this reason, resentment feels entirely justified. We are outraged, as we should be, when evil triumphs and people are unjustly hurt. Anger at injustice isn't sin; it's obligatory. And we're especially outraged if we are the victims! In an article for *Christianity Today*, author Philip Yancey called forgiveness "The Unnatural Act" because everything in us cries out for revenge. Forgiveness is the difficult but crucial choice to not take revenge.

Many people think that forgiveness is acting like the sin didn't happen or it isn't a big deal. Nothing could be farther from the truth. When Christ forgives us, he doesn't excuse our behavior, and he doesn't say that our sins don't matter. They are so serious that the Son of God had to become a man and die to pay the price for them! In the same way, it does no good for us to excuse or minimize sin in our own lives or the lives of others. We need to face it honestly and make the hard choice to apply Christ's payment to those wrongs. Forgiveness is never free. Sin creates a debt, and the debt must be paid. When Christ forgave us, he paid the debt on the cross. In a beautiful description of our freedom, Paul reminded the Colossians that sin had kept them in a debtor's prison. In Roman days, when a person couldn't pay the money he owed, he was thrown into jail and a list of his debts was nailed to the cell door until all the money was paid. Paul tells us, "Christ forgave us all our sins, having canceled the written code, with its regulations, that was against us and that stood opposed to us; he took it away, nailing it to the cross. And having disarmed the powers and authorities, he made a public spectacle of them, triumphing over them by the cross" (Colossians 2:13-15). Jesus doesn't excuse us. He took the list of our debts, every last one of them, and nailed them to his cell door, the cross. His last words on the cross were "Paid in full." That's the assurance we have that every sin we've committed, and every one we'll ever commit, has been completely paid by the blood of Jesus. His forgiveness heals us at our deepest levels. He transforms resentment into gratitude, fear into hope, and anger into kindness.

Only a few paragraphs later in the letter to the Colossians, Paul explains that our experience of God's forgiveness also enables us to express forgiveness to those who have hurt us. To be truly whole, we have to complete the circle of forgiveness by extending God's grace to everyone who has offended us. Paul described our attitude and actions: "Therefore, as God's chosen people, holy and dearly loved, clothe yourselves with compassion, kindness, humility, gentleness and patience. Bear with each other and forgive whatever grievances you may have against one another. Forgive as the Lord forgave you. And over all these virtues put on love, which binds them all together in perfect unity" (Colossians 3:12-14). As Philip Yancey would tell us, forgiveness doesn't just happen. It's a choice we make to move beyond our resentment to obey God and forgive others.

Forgiveness doesn't just let the offender off the hook; it lets *us* off the hook. We no longer are the people who were wronged and who live for revenge. We're free to be the people God wants us to be. Forgiveness opens the door to restoration and reconciliation, but both people need to walk through the door. We forgive unilaterally because God commands it, but trust must be earned. We are foolish to trust someone who hasn't proved he or she is trustworthy. Don't confuse forgiveness and trust.

Choosing to grieve

When we choose to forgive, we face the painful facts of the offense again. Forgiveness, then, always involves grieving the loss experienced from the wound. We may have lost money or possessions when someone stole from us, or we may have lost our childhood or safety when a parent or spouse abused or abandoned us. Every significant offense is a serious loss, and we need to go through the process of grief to heal the hurt and close the wound. The human body has a dozen factors in the clotting and healing process. Spiritually, we have two: forgiving and grieving. If we don't do both of them, we remain bitter, fragile, and furious.

Some of us are quite vocal about our losses, and we tell everybody about them. But others keep our hurts bottled up (in common language, we "stuff" them) until we explode in rage or implode in depression. To experience the healing power of Christ's love and forgiveness, we need to be honest about what we feel. The psalms give us plenty of good examples of brutal honesty. The writers speak of their disappointment, their anger, their despair, and their hurt. Almost always, honesty is the door that leads to a fresh awareness of God's kindness and wisdom, and healing comes. In a beautiful and poignant psalm, Asaph poured out his heart to God to complain that evil people were thriving while he suffered for doing the right thing. He almost yelled, "It's not fair!" His unresolved hurt led to bitterness toward God and people. Finally, he was open to God's perspective. He wrote about the change in his perception:

"*I was senseless and ignorant;*
  I was a brute beast before you.
Yet I am always with you;
  you hold me by my right hand.

You guide me with your counsel,
and afterward you will take me into glory.
Whom have I in heaven but you?
And earth has nothing I desire besides you.
My flesh and my heart may fail,
but God is the strength of my heart
and my portion forever" (Psalm 73:22-26).

The lesson we learn from Asaph is that when we're at our worst, God reaches out and takes our hand to comfort and guide us. Like platelets rushing to the scene of an injury, the blood of Christ opens the floodgates of grace to us when we need it most. When we experience God's kindness and strength in our darkest moments, he transforms us. We stop being resentful, and we realize that he is our greatest treasure.

The aroma of forgiveness and reconciliation

Some of us think that God's grace might work in others' lives, but not in ours. We feel so ashamed for something we've done, and we're sure there can never be any real hope for us. The story of Peter tells us that healing is possible no matter what we've done.

The sacrifice of Jesus is a powerful force that communicates his love to those who feel unlovable, and it assures forgiveness to those whose sins seem insurmountable. One of the most beautiful displays of God's grace in the Bible is found in John's story of Jesus' relationship with Peter before the crucifixion and after the resurrection. At the Last Supper, Jesus told his disciples he was going to be killed. In proud protest, Peter assured Jesus that he would gladly die for him, but Jesus corrected him, "Will you really lay down your life for me? Very truly I tell you, before the rooster crows, you will disown me three times" (John 13:38).

Not much later, Jesus was arrested and was taken to the first of his trials. As Peter waited outside, he kept warm next to a charcoal fire. Three times, people asked Peter if he was one of Jesus' disciples, but each time, he denied it. After the third time, a cock crowed, and Peter wept in shame because he had denied even knowing the One who had been so loving, so faithful, and so true.

After the resurrection, Jesus appeared to individuals and groups on different occasions. During this time, however, Peter gave up on Jesus and his mission. Perhaps his sense of failure caused him to give up hope that he could ever have a role in Christ's kingdom, so Peter took some others fishing. After a long night in the boat with no luck, the men saw someone on the shore. The man told them to cast their nets on the right side, and immediately, they brought in a huge haul of big fish. Peter had seen this a few years before. Instantly, he realized the man on the shore was Jesus. He didn't wait for the other men to row the boat to shore. He jumped in and swam to the beach. He saw that Jesus was cooking fish and bread on a charcoal fire. After they ate, Jesus asked Peter three piercing questions: "Do you love me?" The three questions caused Peter to vividly remember his three denials, and now he was being asked to affirm his love for Jesus in a corresponding way. At that moment, the smell of the charcoal fire on the beach reminded Peter of his worst sins of betrayal—he undoubtedly thought back to the fire weeks earlier when he denied he even knew Jesus. The significance of John's details about the charcoal fires is that God doesn't overlook or minimize our sins. His Spirit reminds us of our worst sins, even as he assures us of his complete forgiveness and restores our relationship with him. For the rest of his life, when Peter talked with people who struggled with shame because of their sin, he could say, "Yeah, I know exactly how you feel. I did a lot worse than that. I denied Jesus, but he forgave me and restored me. If he can do that for me, he can do it for you, too."

Like Peter on the beach with Jesus, when we feel pangs of sorrow and guilt, we don't need to deny those painful feelings or try to medicate them with food, drugs, sex, shopping, or other diversions. The sorrow we feel at that moment is God's hand reaching out to bring us back. The memory of our sin is the smell of the charcoal fire reminding us of our worst sins—at the very moment he assures us that he has completely forgiven us. That kind of sorrow restores spiritual life, frees us from shame, and enflames our love for God more than ever.

Wounded healers

If we think God should keep us from experiencing pain and suffering in this life, we're going to be very disappointed. We have God's assurance that we'll suffer, but he will be with us, heal us, and teach us life's richest lessons so that we can pass those truths along to others who are hurting. And we don't have to walk this path alone. We learn from the Scriptures, by the whisper of the Spirit, and from the support of others who have suffered and experienced God's grace in their darkest hours. As we experience God's healing, we become, in Henri Nouwen's famous phrase, "wounded healers." We are wounded in relationships, and we are healed by them, too.

The saying is true: God never wastes our pain. He weaves his grace into our hurts the way platelets weave fibers to close an open wound. With the wisdom and understanding that comes from experiencing the healing of our deepest hurts, we're able to be the voice, hands, and feet of healing to others. Paul wrote the Corinthians about the transfer of compassion: "Praise be to the God and Father of our Lord Jesus Christ, the Father of compassion and the God of all comfort, who comforts us in all our troubles, so that we can comfort those in any trouble with the comfort we ourselves have received from God. For just as the sufferings of Christ flow over into our lives, so also through Christ our comfort overflows" (2 Corinthians 1:3-5).

If you don't know what Paul was talking about, then first you probably need to experience some healing in your life. Find the courage to be honest with God. Like the psalmists, pour out your heart to him, and trust him to meet you in the darkest place of pain. But don't go through it alone. Find someone who understands, who has walked this road before, and who doesn't try to "fix" your problems too quickly. Sadly, the body of Christ too often is a place where unhealed hurts lead us to lash out in anger and gossip behind people's backs, causing even more wounds. But it only takes one courageous person to say, "Enough is enough. I choose to love, forgive, and heal, and I want to be a source of healing for people in my community." Jonathan was that person for King David, and Barnabas was that person for Paul. We don't have to have all the answers; we just need to let God use our own stories of healing to encourage others to take the next step in their own journeys. Some will think we've lost our minds, but a few will take our hands and walk with us.

Dallas Theological Seminary Professor Ramesh Richard has said that the deepest wounds we experience in the first part of our lives often become the platform of our greatest ministry for the rest of our lives. That's true of me, and it's true for countless others. The deep hurt I experienced when my mother died threatened to overwhelm me, but in time, God used the pain to give me compassion for others who suffer. I doubt I'd be a doctor or a pastor today if I hadn't endured those hurts and if God hadn't used them to touch my life so deeply.

A hymn by Edward Mote tells of the glory of Christ's forgiveness and his comfort in times of suffering:

"My hope is built on nothing less
than Jesus' blood and righteousness.

I dare not trust the sweetest frame,
but wholly lean on Jesus' name.

Refrain:
On Christ the solid rock I stand,
all other ground is sinking sand;
all other ground is sinking sand.

When Darkness veils his lovely face,
I rest on his unchanging grace.
In every high and stormy gale,
my anchor holds within the veil.

His oath, his covenant, his blood
supports me in the whelming flood.
When all around my soul gives way,
he then is all my hope and stay.

When he shall come with trumpet sound,
O may I then in him be found!
Dressed in his righteousness alone,
faultless to stand before the throne!" [20]

Platelets in our bloodstream do a marvelous work of identifying wounds and rushing to begin the healing process. Beyond our ability to see with unaided eyes, they perform a series of complex maneuvers to plug the hole and stop the flow of blood, saving our lives. They sacrifice themselves to heal our hurts, just as Jesus sacrificed himself

---

20 "My Hope is Built," lyrics by Edward Mote, music by William Bradbury.

to heal our spiritual and emotional wounds. His grace is readily available to reach all our hurts—on the surface where we see them and hidden deep below. The process of healing a cut or a scrape takes time and patience, but it heals beautifully. Sometimes, a wound is so deep and ugly that doctors have to cut out diseased tissue so that healthy tissue can heal. It's painful, and it often leaves a scar, but the scar is a sign of healing. Occasionally, God has to do surgery in our lives to cut out diseased, necrotic attitudes and misperceptions that can't heal. God is a skilled surgeon who cuts quickly and deeply to get to the infected area. This kind of spiritual surgery and the healing process always involve honesty, forgiveness, and grief. In our lives, forgiving is a choice we can make in an instant, but grieving is a process that often takes a lot of time, especially if the wound is deep and prolonged. But in time, healing comes. We can count on it.

Think about it...

1.   How do platelets respond when we are injured?

2. Is a scab a sign of a wound or of healing? Explain your answer.

3. Why is forgiveness (both experiencing it and expressing it) essential to spiritual, emotional, and relational healing?

4. Explain the connection between forgiveness and grief.

5. How does the story of Peter, Jesus, and the charcoal fires give us courage to confess our sins and experience Christ's forgiveness?

6. What are the lessons you have learned (or are learning or need to learn) from the healing of your deepest wounds?

Two Meals, One Memory

"Here is the truly fantastic assertion that through the shedding of Jesus' blood in death God was taking the initiative to establish a new pact or 'covenant' with his people, one of the greatest promises of which would be the forgiveness of sinners."

—John R. W. Stott

In our relatively safe and sanitized world, it's difficult for us to grasp the explosive power of the emotions in the slave quarters in Egypt at the first Passover and over a millennia later in the Upper Room at the ultimate Passover. We're so familiar with these events that they, well, bore us. We need to go back and recapture some of the pathos of those pivotal times in spiritual history. When we genuinely understand the nature of God and the message of the gospel, we're either astonished or enraged—nothing in between. The two meals God instituted are both based in blood, and they share a common memory.

Escape from Death

The people of God had lost hope. For over 400 years, they had cruelly suffered as slaves in a foreign land. Centuries before, God had given Abraham a solemn promise to bless them and make them a blessing to all the nations of the world, but during the years of spiritual drought, the promise looked like an empty one. Where was God? How could he have let this happen to his people? Then, through strange and wonderful circumstances, a man from Pharaoh's own court became their champion. Moses stood up for them, and he even killed an Egyptian who was beating one of their people. But the flicker of hope for quick deliverance quickly vanished when he was exiled to the backside of nowhere. For forty more years, the people struggled each day under the lash to build cities for people who despised them. Day after day, they suffered, bled, and died physically, but even worse, they felt abandoned by God.

One day, Moses reappeared in Pharaoh's court. He looked different. Sure, he was a lot older, but he had a fire in his eyes no one had seen in generations. It was the fire of hope. He confronted the most powerful man on the planet and demanded that he let the people of Israel go free. When Pharaoh refused, God began making, to use the Godfather's famous line, "an offer he couldn't refuse." He sent plague after plague: turning the Nile into blood, a swarm of frogs, lice, flies, the death of livestock, painful boils, hail that killed all the crops and the remaining cattle and sheep, locusts, and darkness. But Pharaoh still said no.

The people of God watched all this in amazement. No one had stood up for them for so long, and now God was performing miracles to set them free. The obstinate Pharaoh, however, wasn't cooperating with God's plan. Now, the stage was set for one more demonstration of God's awesome power. He was going to send the angel of death across the land to kill the first-born son in every family. The devastation would wreck the culture, but God gave the Hebrews a way to protect their sons from certain death. He told them, "On that same night I will pass through Egypt and strike down every firstborn—both men and animals—and I will bring judgment on all the gods of Egypt. I am the LORD. The blood will be a sign for you on the houses where you are; and when I see the blood, I will pass over you. No destructive plague will touch you when I strike Egypt" (Exodus 12:12-13). He gave them clear, detailed instructions about preparing bread without yeast and slaughtering an unblemished lamb as a sacrifice.

Moses told the leaders of the people, "Go at once and select the animals for your families and slaughter the Passover lamb. Take a bunch of hyssop, dip it into the blood in the basin and put some of the blood on the top and on both sides of the doorframe. Not one of you shall go out the door of his house until morning. When the LORD goes through the land to strike down the Egyptians, he will see the blood on the top and sides of the doorframe and will pass over that doorway, and he will not permit the destroyer to enter your houses and strike you down" (Exodus 12:21-23).

That night, as they listened to wails of sorrow from homes across Egypt, every Hebrew family that had the lamb's blood on its doorframe was spared. That night, they ate a feast of unleavened bread, herbs, and roasted lamb, giving thanks to God for sparing their lives. They were sure none of them would ever forget the horror of death and the joy of deliverance they experienced that night. They would never wonder if resistance to God's will was serious or not—it had cost Pharaoh, the Egyptians, and any unbelieving Hebrews their first-born sons' lives. And they'd never question God's ability to forgive and restore them. After the death and destruction of that night,

Pharaoh told the people to leave, and the people of Egypt gave the slaves gold and other gifts as they left for the Promised Land. They were free, but it had cost the life of an unblemished lamb for every family, sacrificed so that sons might live.

The events of that night are the seminal truth in the history of the Jewish people. From that day, they have celebrated the angel of death passing over their houses when he saw the blood on the door-frames. Passover is the most solemn and joyful event in the Jewish calendar.

Each year, the date has been determined by the first full moon after the spring equinox. It is followed by seven days of the Feast of Unleavened Bread. Over the centuries, an elaborate and meaningful ritual, called the *seder*, was established to help Jewish people remember God's deliverance on that first Passover night. Unleavened bread reminds them that the people had to prepare the dinner in haste, so they didn't have time to let their bread rise. Bitter herbs remind them of the bitterness of slavery in Egypt. Four cups of wine relate to different parts of the story and the celebration. Four questions reflect on the events and the meaning of the Passover night. Lamb is prepared very carefully and is the center of the feast. The Hallel, Psalms 113 to 118, is sung at the end, with the concluding cry, "Next year in Jerusalem!" Every part of the Passover meal is significant. It speaks of the glorious past of God's deliverance from Egypt, the current connections with each other as the family of God, and their hope to be in the center of God's purposes and presence in the future.

Passover isn't just a lecture; it's a family feast. People sitting around the table don't just hear with their ears. They engage every sensory organ to see and hold the food, taste and smell it, hear the answers to the questions, and sing the songs. Active participation heightens the senses of every person at the table. The children aren't

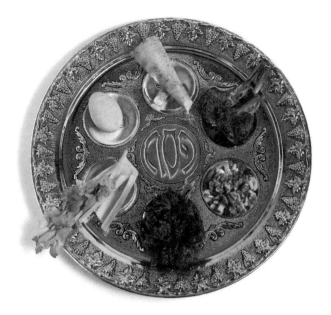

Figure 10. The Passover meal.

excluded. In fact, children have an important role in the seder. A parent or grandparent often prompts the youngest child to ask the traditional questions, beginning with the words, "Mah Nishtana Ha-Leila HaZeh?" ("Why is this night different from all other nights?") People around the table then discuss the significance of the elements of the meal.

Family connections mean everything in the Jewish culture. Years ago, I treated the son of one of the leading rabbis in Chicago. The young man had leukemia, and he was completely cured. At the end of several years of therapy, the rabbi and his son came to see me. The young man looked at me and said, "I owe you my life. Because you gave my life back to me, I am obligated by Jewish custom to invest my life to help others, and I'm glad to do it." The young man attended a rabbinic college and became a rabbi so he could teach others about God. He got married and began serving in a synagogue. About a year ago, he called me. His voice was choked with tears as he told me that he and his wife were expecting a son. He realized that he could easily have died, but God used modern medicine to rescue him and give him his life back. And now, he had the joy of bringing a new generation into the world. To him and his whole family, it was God's miracle. Because God used me, they consider me part of their family. It was, in fact, a miracle wrought by the incredible healing power of blood!

Throughout history, the Jewish race has been hounded from cities and nations, attacked by governments and hotheaded individuals, and most significantly, murdered by the millions in Hitler's gas chambers during World War II. These people, though, have never forgotten the first Passover when they were oppressed as slaves in a foreign land, and God directed them to put the blood of an unblemished lamb on their doorframes to protect them from evil and free them from oppression. Today, it means as much to them as it has meant during the past three millennia. Even in their darkest time, blood brought freedom. The sacrifice and the feast bind them together and give them compassion for strangers and others in need.

In the Upper Room

Two thousand years ago in Palestine, a carpenter's son celebrated Passover with his family. As his father killed the costly, unblemished lamb, Jesus caught a glimpse of his future. As they ate the meal and celebrated the feast, he looked forward to that day when he would eat it with his followers the night before he, the perfect Lamb, was slaughtered for all of us. And he may have thought about a time in the distant future when another feast will be held, the Marriage Feast of the Lamb, when people from every tongue, tribe, and nation will gather in God's eternal kingdom to celebrate the Lamb who was slain for them.

When Jesus began his public ministry, John the Baptist pointed to him and pronounced, "Behold, the Lamb of God who takes away the sins of the world!" (John 1:29) For three and a half years, Jesus lived, taught, healed, and modeled spiritual life and forgiveness. During those years, he baffled people by accepting tax collectors and prostitutes but enraging the respected, established religious leaders. He turned things upside down! In his interactions, he often told people he healed not to tell anyone. Why would he make a request like this? Because, he said, "My time has not yet come." The term "my time" refers to his death. If word spread too broadly that he was the Messiah, the people might get in the way of his ultimate plan: not to live a glorious life, but to die a glorious death.

When he entered Jerusalem the Sunday before his arrest, Jesus knew that his time had come at last. He allowed the people to proclaim him as king, and they shouted "Hosanna!" as he entered the city on the back of a colt. During the week, he argued with the religious leaders again about the meaning of spiritual life, threw the merchants out of the temple, and taught his followers important truths about the coming kingdom. On Thursday night, he prepared to have his final meal with the Twelve.

When they arrived in the Upper Room to celebrate Passover, there was no servant to wash their feet. Certainly, no self-respecting Jew, and especially no one who expected to be an official in Jesus' cabinet when he became king, would stoop to wash the others' feet. Instead, they argued about who would be the greatest! To their shock and horror, the Lord of Glory took off his robe, picked up a towel, and assumed the role of the lowest servant by washing their feet. He explained that greatness didn't come from positions but by stooping to serve. He announced that one of them would betray him, and in an almost comic scene, they all wondered if they were the one he was talking about. But one of them knew. Judas had already made his deal with the devil to betray Jesus.

At some point in the Passover dinner, Jesus stopped, took a piece of bread in his hands, gave thanks, and broke it. As he passed it around to the men, he told them, "Take and eat; this is my body."

When each of them had eaten a piece of bread, he picked up a cup of wine, gave thanks, and passed it to the men, saying, "Drink from it, all of you. This is my blood of the covenant, which is poured out for many for the forgiveness of sins" (Matthew 26:26-28).

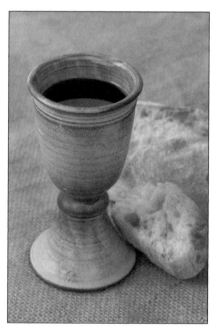

Figure 11. The cup and the bread.

What was Jesus talking about when he talked about "the covenant" in his blood? Six hundred years before, during a time of calamity for the nation of Israel, Jeremiah had predicted that God would someday inaugurate a new covenant. The old one had begun at Mt. Sinai, and was steeped in the blood of bulls and goats as offerings for sin. The new one would be categorically different. Jeremiah reported:

" 'The time is coming,' declares the LORD,

    'when I will make a new covenant

    with the house of Israel

    and with the house of Judah.

 It will not be like the covenant

    I made with their forefathers

    when I took them by the hand

    to lead them out of Egypt,

    because they broke my covenant,

    though I was a husband to them,'

    declares the LORD.

'This is the covenant I will make with the house of Israel

    after that time,' declares the LORD.

    'I will put my law in their minds

    and write it on their hearts.

    I will be their God,

    and they will be my people.

 No longer will a man teach his neighbor,

    or a man his brother, saying, "Know the LORD,"

    because they will all know me,

    from the least of them to the greatest,'

    declares the LORD.

    For I will forgive their wickedness

    and will remember their sins no more' "

    (Jeremiah 31:31-34).

The central, defining characteristic of the new covenant would be the blood shed by the Lamb of God to pay for the sins of the world. Though Jesus and his disciples celebrated the Passover on Thursday evening, the Passover lambs were actually sacrificed the next afternoon—at the time he was dying on the cross. To explain how the Passover could be celebrated on two dates, Professor John R. W. Stott observes, "Either the Pharisees and Sadducees were using alternative calendars, which differed from each other by a day, or there were so many pilgrims in Jerusalem for the festival (perhaps as many as 100,000) that the Galileans killed their lambs on Thursday and ate them that evening, while the Judeans observed the celebration a day later."[21] Another explanation is offered by Maret H. Dinsmore in his book, *What Really Happened When Christ Died.* He suggests that the Jewish calendar observed multiple Sabbaths all in a row.

All the sacrifices on the Jewish altars for all those centuries were only a shadow of the supreme sacrifice. The God of the universe had become a man and lived a sinless life so that he could be the spotless Lamb slain for all time for all people. Five times in the book of Hebrews, the writer tells us that Jesus' sacrifice was given "once for all," never again to be repeated because it is completely sufficient for all time.

The new covenant shocked the sensibilities of the people who thought they could manage and control God by following rules. The Pharisees and Sadducees had multiplied the laws to be sure they could control their behavior and prove they were worthy of God's acceptance. When Jesus walked among them, though, he blew their expectations into the creek! He partied with Levi, a tax collector,

---

21   John R. W. Stott, *The Cross of Christ,* (Intervarsity Press, Downers Grove, Illinois, 2006), p. 74.

touched a leper, healed crippled people on the Sabbath, and generally told the religious leaders that their way of relating to God simply didn't work. They were furious with him. The fiercest debates in the gospels were between Jesus and these rigid, demanding, legalistic leaders. Over and over again, Jesus tried to explain to them that he was going to make everything new. At one point, he told them two parables with a single point: "No one tears a patch from a new garment and sews it on an old one. If he does, he will have torn the new garment, and the patch from the new will not match the old. And no one pours new wine into old wineskins. If he does, the new wine will burst the skins, the wine will run out, and the wineskins will be ruined. No, new wine must be poured into new wineskins. And no one after drinking old wine wants the new, for he says, 'The old is better' " (Luke 5:36-39). The new covenant of grace required a new garment and new wineskins. Old habits of law, performance, and fear simply aren't part of Christ's new order.

The language of the Last Supper has become common for most of us, but it certainly wasn't familiar to the people of that day. In John's gospel, we read of a series of miraculous events earlier in Jesus' ministry, and then a hot contest of wills. Jesus fed five thousand men (probably about twenty thousand people, including women and children) with a boy's sack lunch. After he had instructed his disciples to sail across the lake, a storm frightened them. To their surprise, they saw Jesus walking to them on the water. When they reached the other shore, a throng of people who had eaten lunch with him came to see if he could do any more tricks. They didn't understand the significance of the sign he had given them, and he corrected their misperceptions. The argument went back and forth. They wanted bread and miracles; Jesus offered them a relationship with himself and eternal life. Finally, he told them, "I'm the bread of life." When they didn't seem to understand or care, he announced, "I tell you the truth, unless you eat the flesh of the Son of Man and drink his blood, you have no life in you. Whoever eats my flesh and drinks my blood has eternal life, and I will raise him up at the last day. For my flesh is real food and my blood is real drink. Whoever eats my flesh and drinks my blood remains in me, and I in him" (John 6:53-56).

Jesus could hardly have said anything more shocking or offensive. The people were outraged and horrified, and the thousands melted away until only the Twelve were left. Jesus' message that day in Capernaum, though, sounds very much like the institution of the new covenant at the Last Supper. In fact, it's exactly the same. The point Jesus was making to the crowd that day and to his disciples in the Upper Room is that following him is a personal commitment. We don't just learn about him or join a movement. We become, as Peter describes it, "partakers of the divine nature." Countless people in our churches know the Bible stories, sing the songs, and attend committee meetings, but that's not the essence of the new covenant in his blood. In it, we eat, we drink, we taste his kindness and love, we sense the strength that comes from his Spirit living in us, and we delight in a banquet of knowing him. I can't eat his body and drink his blood for you. I can only do it for myself. Parents can bring their children to the table, but the children must ultimately decide if they want to eat and drink of Christ.

When we taste Jesus, the doorway of heaven opens, and we enter into the very presence of God. At the moment of Jesus' death at Calvary outside Jerusalem, a miracle happened across town. Matthew records the event: "At that moment the curtain of the temple was torn in two from top to bottom" (Matthew 27:51). The temple wasn't like today's churches. It had several courts, like the ones for women and Gentiles, who weren't allowed to come into the temple itself. Inside the temple, the most sacred place was the holy of holies, which housed the ark of the covenant holding Aaron's rod and the tablets of the Ten Commandments. The high priest entered this room once a year on Yom Kippur, the Day of Atonement, to offer sacrifice to God. A heavy curtain sixty feet high enclosed this small room. The Jewish historian Josephus reported that the veil was four inches thick, so strong that horses tied to each side couldn't pull it apart. At the moment Jesus breathed his last breath, the veil was miraculously ripped from top to bottom. This signified that the blood of Jesus opened the door for anyone who believes in him to enter the presence of God.

How often do we need to remember the sacrifice of Christ? When Paul explained the significance and process of the Lord's Table to the Corinthians, he told them, "For whenever you eat this bread and drink this cup, you proclaim the Lord's death until he comes" (1 Corinthians 11:26). Many churches celebrate the Last Supper once a week, some once a month, and sadly, some celebrate it rarely if ever. There are some faith traditions, though, that understand Paul's words to mean that every time they eat, they should take a few minutes to reflect on the sacrifice of Christ and the new covenant in his blood. I'm not sure we ever get tired of thinking about the God of glory humbling himself to die for us. That's a message I need to hear several times a day.

Eucharist

Another term for our celebration of the Last Supper is the Eucharist, which means thanksgiving. When we realize what Jesus has done for us, we're overwhelmed with gratitude. If we have an ounce of self-awareness, we quickly realize that we don't deserve his love, forgiveness, and kindness. We are selfish people, and apart from the grace of God, we richly deserve the sentence of eternal death and hell. Two of the most beautiful words in the Bible are "but God." When Paul described our moral depravity and sinfulness to the Ephesians, he said we are spiritually dead, hopeless, and helpless. Even our good deeds to try to prove we are worthy of him are a stench to God. Then Paul says, "But God, being rich in mercy, because of His great love with which He loved us, even when we were dead in our transgressions, made us alive together with Christ (by grace you have been saved), and raised us up with Him, and seated us with Him in the heavenly places in Christ Jesus, so that in the ages to come He might show the surpassing riches of His grace in kindness toward us in Christ Jesus" (Ephesians 2:4-7). I love that last verse. It tells me a lot about God's heart. He doesn't sit back with arms folded waiting for me to sin so that he can condemn me. Instead, he longs to show me more of his grace, unfolding in multitudes of kindness and love for the rest of time and eternity.

When we feel oppressed like slaves, we can remember that the blood on the doorframes instituted an exodus led by the first Moses, and we now follow Jesus, the second Moses, in a new exodus out of sin and slavery to freedom in God's kingdom. We haven't earned this privilege; it's a free gift. Every time we realize how little we deserve God's love but how freely he gives it, we are humbled to the dust, and our hearts sing with joy.

Also, when we realize what the new covenant cost Jesus, we appreciate even more how he suffered for us. He didn't have to go to the cross. No one made him undergo the awful pain—nothing but love prompted him to endure and spill his blood. We talk a lot in the church about the importance of obedience, but I'm afraid some people misunderstand. They think that obedience is a way to earn points with God, but that's not it at all. We obey because we are already blessed, not to be blessed. We long to please the one who loves us and died to save us. As we are overwhelmed with this reality, we become truly zealous for Christ. Bishop J. C. Ryle wrote about the compelling nature of genuine zeal:

"Zeal in religion is a burning desire to please God, to do His will, and to advance His glory in the world in every possible way. It is a desire which no man feels by nature—which the Spirit puts in the heart of every believer when he is converted. . . . A zealous man is preeminently a man of one thing. It is not enough to say that he is earnest, hearty, uncompromising, thoroughgoing, wholehearted, fervent in spirit. He only sees one thing, he cares for one thing, he lives for one thing, he is swallowed up in one thing; and that one thing is to please God. Whether he lives, or whether he dies—whether he has health, or whether he has sickness—whether he is rich, or whether he is poor—whether he pleases man, or whether he gives offense . . . for all this the zealous man cares nothing at all."[22]

Above all, those who continually feast on the body and blood of Jesus are grateful people. They can hardly imagine how they could be so blessed to be forgiven, loved, and accepted when they deserve just the opposite. Every day is like winning the lottery and getting out of jail! An accurate view of the sacrifice of Christ corrects our thoughts and changes our attitudes. Instead of demanding our way, we become thankful, humble, gentle, and strong. But grace never makes us passive. Instead, gratitude and humility take us down the path toward God's purposes for us and for the world. In his book,

---

22 Bishop J. C. Ryle, *Practical Religion*, 1959, p. 130.

Uprising: A Revolution of the Soul, author and pastor Erwin McManus observes, "We are called to no less than the very attitude of Jesus who humbled Himself and gave His life on our behalf. Submission unites us to the mission."[23] The message of grace isn't reserved for perfect people. Over and over again, Jesus reached out to broken people to touch their darkest sins, deepest wounds, and crippling fears, and he transformed them. Today, we need his touch. We long for him to reach into our secret sins, our bitterness and pride, our nagging doubts, our strained relationships, and our discouragement and depression. The message of the two meals leads to a strong, compelling memory that the blood of Jesus meets us where we are, frees us from bondage, and opens the door to the most glorious freedom and purpose life can offer.

One of my favorite hymns is "At Calvary" by William R. Newell. Let the message capture your heart and remind you of the body and blood of Jesus.

"Years I spent in vanity and pride,

Caring not my Lord was crucified,

Knowing not it was for me He died on Calvary.

Refrain:

Mercy there was great, and grace was free;

Pardon there was multiplied to me;

There my burdened soul found liberty at Calvary.

---

23 Erwin McManus, *Uprising: A Revolution of the Soul,* (Thomas Nelson Publishers, Nashville, 2003).

By God's Word at last my sin I learned;

Then I trembled at the law I'd spurned,

Till my guilty soul imploring turned to Calvary.

Now I've given to Jesus everything,

Now I gladly own Him as my King,

Now my raptured soul can only sing of Calvary!

Oh, the love that drew salvation's plan!

Oh, the grace that brought it down to man!

Oh, the mighty gulf that God did span at Calvary!" [24]

The Beauty of Communion

In many ways, God works in our lives the way Jesus instituted the Last Supper. He blesses us, he breaks us through difficulties, and then with new wisdom and compassion, he gives us to others to impart grace to them. In the same way, when we drink the love and grace of Jesus, we are filled up and pour it out to nourish others.

When we participate in the body and blood of Jesus, we do it corporately. We don't give ourselves the elements; someone gives them to us. And when we offer the elements to each other, we extend grace in its fullest measure. Our participation in the meal, then, is the reaffirmation of our love for one another, our commitment to each other's best, and our willingness to forgive, to bear each other's burdens, and help each other grow.

---

24 "At Calvary," Words and Music by William R Newell, 1868-1956, & Daniel B. Towner, 1850-1919.

The two meals we find in the Bible are tremendously important. They remind us of sacrifice and freedom, and they reinforce the most important payment ever made: the blood of Jesus for our sins. When Jesus tells us to remember, he's not referring only to *the events* surrounding his death on the cross. Even more, he wants us to remember *the significance* of those events. His blood was shed for helpless men and women who were lost, "without God and without hope in the world," but Jesus paid the price to win us back and give us hope.

Think about it...

1. What do you think it would have felt like and sounded like if your family had participated in the first Passover, putting blood on the doorframe of your house, eating the meal, and listening to the wails of families that lost sons?

2. Why was it significant that Jesus washed the disciples feet before he told them about the new covenant in his blood?

3. Is there a Christian faith without the blood of Jesus sacrificed for our sins? Why or why not?

4. What are a few reasons some people may know a lot about Jesus and the crucifixion but not apply it to their sins?

5. In what way is grasping the significance of the new covenant in Jesus' blood even better than winning the lottery and getting out of jail?

6. Is Bishop Ryle's description of a zealous person attractive to you? Why or why not?

7. What can you do to make your participation in the Lord's Supper more meaningful to you? What have you learned from this chapter that might help you?

6

Living in the Shadow of the Cross

" None of us feels the true love of God till we realize how wicked we are. But you can't teach people that—they have to learn by experience."

—Dorothy L. Sayers

A pastor dryly noted, "We've been able to accomplish something Jesus' enemies could never do: we've made him look boring and unappealing." Countless people sit in churches each Sunday without the slightest flicker of emotion—neither hope nor fear, neither dreams nor dreads, and neither delight or sorrow. They seem to have very little grasp of the wonder of God's magnificent grace that transforms lives.

The problem, though, isn't quite as simple as that. Others come to church regularly—we might even say, religiously. They've grown up hearing all the "Thou shalts" and even more, the "Thou shalt nots." To them, the Christian life is an enormous scorecard. Their goal is to make sure they have all their boxes checked, and if a few aren't checked, they hope no one notices. They feel distant from God, but they expect him to come through for them because they've "done so much for him."

A third type of person sits in the pews each Sunday. They've been exposed to the misguided teaching that promises God will give them whatever they want. They see the Lord of glory as a cosmic vending machine. They delight in hearing stories about him providing wealth, health, and happiness, and they're sure their ship is coming in soon. After a while, if the vending machine lets them down, they become deeply discouraged and may even walk away from God.

Children of God

We will only learn to relate to God in a rich and real way if we understand how the death of Christ secures for us a vibrant relationship with God. We don't have a business relationship with God. We are his children. In *Knowing God*, author and professor J. I. Packer observes, "What is a Christian? The question can be answered in many ways, but the richest answer I know is that a Christian is one who has God as Father. . . . If you want to know how well a person understands Christianity, find out how much he makes of the thought of being God's child, and having God as his Father. If this is not the thought that prompts and controls his worship and prayers and his whole outlook on life, it means that he does not understand Christianity very well at all."[25] A sculptor may make a bronze statue, or an artist may paint a beautiful picture, but neither of these

---

25 Packer, *Knowing God*, pp. 181f.

created objects actually has the inherent nature of the creator. A child, though, has the DNA of her parents. At the moment we were born again, many things happened to us. Our address changed from "the domain of darkness" to the "kingdom of Christ," and we were "born again." God put his Spirit inside us, and we were made children of God. We were instantly changed, and paradoxically, we are continually changed until we see him face to face.

When asked to summarize the teaching of the New Testament, Dr. Packer put it in three words: "adoption through propitiation." This pregnant phrase tells us about the true nature of our relationship with God, and it explains the cost paid to secure it. Propitiation isn't a term we hear very often, but the concept is woven throughout the Scriptures. In some versions of the Bible, the term is translated as "atonement." It means to satisfy the righteous wrath of God, and it is always associated with the blood of Christ. For some of us, the idea of "wrath" seems to be so, well, politically incorrect. Our culture values tolerance: what's true for you may not be true for me, so let's not judge each other. The Bible, however, doesn't mince words. It says that apart from Christ, we richly deserve the wrath of God, which is poured out against sin. In fact, sinners "store up wrath for the day of wrath" (Ephesians 2:3). In our day, we also fail to appreciate the holiness of God. We treat him like he's our buddy, but he "dwells in unapproachable light." The Bible says that the right response to God's holiness is fear. We can redefine this fear as awe and reverence, but when people came face to face with angels, they were terrified! How awesome is it to realize that we live each moment in the presence of the Creator of the universe whose holiness is an "unquenchable fire."

To the degree that we minimize the seriousness of sin and the holiness of God, we'll underestimate the glory of grace. Those who are truly aware of their wickedness desperately need and greatly appreciate God's magnificent grace shown most vividly in the sacrificial death of Christ to pay for our sins.

Some of us—in fact, some who attend church most regularly—believe that we can do enough good deeds and avoid some of the big sins, and thereby twist God's arm so that he accepts us. Self-effort makes us our own saviors, and we're not qualified for that role. No matter how many laws we keep, how much money we give, how little we cuss, and how squeaky clean we appear to be, our hearts are still rotten to the core. Like the Pharisees, we are "whitewashed tombs," clean on the outside but dead on the inside. Following a list of rules doesn't solve the problem. Paul told the Romans, "But now a righteousness from God, apart from law, has been made known, to which the Law and the Prophets testify. This righteousness from God comes through faith in Jesus Christ to all who believe. There is no difference, for all have sinned and fall short of the glory of God, and are justified freely by his grace through the redemption that came by Christ Jesus. God presented him as a sacrifice of atonement, through faith in his blood" (Romans 3:21-25).

Everything in the Old Testament pointed to the One who would come, fulfill the law, and provide the final sacrifice for sin. Jesus didn't offer a lamb to God; he *is* the lamb. He didn't ask a priest to offer it; he *is* the high priest. He didn't hope a king would inaugurate a new kingdom; he *is* the king of glory.

We may not say it out loud, but some of us wonder if the death of Jesus wasn't just a big mistake. He was a great teacher, a noble leader, and a friend to the down and out. Surely, we suppose, his death was one of the biggest blunders in history. If he had lived, maybe he could have taught us even better how to love each other.

No, he taught us well enough, but the primary reason he came wasn't to teach us how to love people better. That's part of it, but only part. The primary reason he came was to die. From the beginning, sacrificing his life and pouring out his blood was the Father's plan and the ultimate purpose of Christ. Many times in conversations with his followers, he told them he was going to be killed. It certainly wasn't a shock to him when it happened—finally, his time had come. Crucifixion is perhaps the cruelest form of execution the world has ever known. After Jesus' back was flayed open, exposing the bone and flesh, large nails were hammered through his wrists and feet into the beams, and then, suspended above the earth for all the world to see his shame, his weight hung on those nails. Matthew tells us Jesus "cried out in a loud voice." In other words, he screamed in agony. He yelled, "My God, my God, why have you forsaken me?" (Matthew 26:46) Some scholars have noted that Jesus surely must have said those words because no writer of fiction would put such a cry of despair in the mouth of someone who was purported to be the leader of a new religious movement. At that moment, the agony Jesus experienced wasn't primarily physical; it was spiritual. All the sins of everyone the world has ever known and will ever know was poured out on him. To shoulder this staggering burden of paying for all sin, he had to be separated from the Father. He experienced an eternity of hell for every person, including you and me.

Who did Jesus die for? Was it people who are "pretty good" and need only a little help to make them acceptable to God? No, there aren't any like that. He died for people who are enemies of God, totally self-absorbed, with hearts darkened by sin, and who try to cover up their rotten hearts by wearing a smile in public—people like us.

Just before he died, Luke tells us that Jesus screamed again. His last words were, "Father, into your hands I commit my spirit" (Luke

23:46). At that moment, the reason for every lamb being slain for the Passover was finished—the Lamb of God had been slaughtered.

What did Jesus' death accomplish for us? There are many things, but the one we're examining here is that it changed the nature of our relationship with God. The status as sons that we could never have acquired on our own was a free gift of God's magnificent grace. Those who accept his death to pay for their sins are immediately transformed and adopted into his family. Paul explained to the Romans, "And if the Spirit of him who raised Jesus from the dead is living in you, he who raised Christ from the dead will also give life to your mortal bodies through his Spirit, who lives in you. . . . For you did not receive a spirit that makes you a slave again to fear, but you received the Spirit of sonship. And by him we cry, 'Abba, Father.' The Spirit himself testifies with our spirit that we are God's children" (Romans 8:11, 15-16).

In the ancient world, it was common for wealthy Romans to adopt an adult to inherit the family fortune and carry on the family name. In the classic movie, *Ben Hur,* the slave, Judah Ben Hur, was adopted by the Roman general Arias. Ben Hur was a galley slave, but during a battle, he escaped and saved Arias' life. In gratitude, Arias adopted him, loved him, and gave him all the benefits of being his own child.

Of course, you and I did nothing to earn our adoption, but the new wealth and status Ben Hur enjoyed as the adopted son of Arias parallel our riches in God's grace and our status of being the King's children. The closeness Arias and Ben Hur developed is similar to the relationship we can have with God. Paul encourages us to call God "Abba, Father." Abba means Daddy, a term of intimacy and endearment. God didn't rescue us and then leave us alone. He saved us because he loves us: dearly, intimately, and tenderly. Jesus called

God "Father," and we are invited to call him that name, too. In her encouraging book, *Into Abba's Arms*, Sandy Wilson writes:

"Jesus not only addressed God as Father, he invites us to address God in this shockingly personal and intimate way. How that unprecedented intimacy with God must have scandalized the theologians who heard Jesus teach! After all, our Savior intro-duced an astounding premise: When we approach God, we can come to him as a child runs to a loving daddy. . . . We don't usually think of being tenderly embraced by kings, warriors, or judges, and Scripture portrays God in those terms, too. But a faithful, loving daddy—ah, that's a different story."[26]

When our hearts are gripped with the reality that we are sons and daughters of the King, and that our new status as his children was bought by the blood of Jesus, we never look at life the same again. We have a new affection for God. We respond to his great love by loving him in return. We long to honor him, and we delight in talking about his goodness and grace. We also recognize his authority as our Father. We may have had a rotten dad—absent or abusive—but in contrast, God has proven that he is supremely trustworthy. When he speaks, we don't rebel like an angry teenager. We listen, and we're glad to follow his leading, even if we're not sure where his leading will take us. Obeying Someone who loves us so much isn't a grind; it's a delight.

The nature of human blood is a beautiful metaphor of God's love for us as his children. When my daughters were babies and little girls, Susan and I did all kinds of things for them that they didn't

---

26 Sandy Wilson, *Into Abba's Arms,* (Tyndale, Wheaton, Illinois, 1998), p. 62.

even realize. Of course, they knew that we were nourishing them with food, eliminating waste by changing their diapers and giving them baths, protecting them from harm, and soothing them when they scraped their knees or experienced disappointments. These are, as we've seen, the properties of red cells, white cells, and platelets, and they are the characteristics of loving, attentive, strong parents—and God is the ultimate parent. Good parents think nothing of giving their lives for their children. They step in front of a truck, donate a kidney, dive into frigid waters, and do anything and everything it takes to save their child's life. When Jesus died on the cross, he performed the greatest parental act of sacrificial love the world has ever seen. Theologians call it *substitutionary atonement*. We deserved death, but Jesus took our place, paid our penalty, and rescued us.

When we stand at the foot of the cross and look at Jesus, we realize that Christianity isn't just a good moral philosophy. It's that, but it's far more. It's not just a set of rules that make life better if we follow them. It's that, but it's much more. The heart of the gospel is a payment made in blood that demonstrates the depth of God's love, the height of his commitment to us, and the breadth of his strength to provide everything we need for life and godliness. We don't obey to get leverage so God will bless us. We obey because we've been so blessed that our hearts explode with pure joy and thankfulness. We want to please the One who cares for us so much. The love of God is written in Jesus' blood.

Our Treasure

On July 20, 1985, Mel Fisher stood on the deck of his salvage boat in the waters off the Florida Keys; for twenty years, he had been searching for a ship called the Atocha, a Spanish galleon loaded with treasure. It had sunk in a hurricane early in the 17th century.

He and his crew had found some gold bars near the site where they searched that day, and they were hopeful they'd find more—much more. Fisher had quite an investment in the venture. He mortgaged everything he had and borrowed much more to keep the operation going. Ten years before, his son and another diver had drowned during the search. Financially, relationally, and professionally, Fisher was "all in."

As he watched from the decks, his crew rigged up the pipe to blow sand away from the sea floor, and then some divers went down to see if anything had been uncovered. Fisher looked at the bubbles from the scuba tanks as he had done countless times before, and then suddenly, one of the divers exploded to the surface, ripped off his mask and yelled, "It's here! We've found the main pile!" As the sand cleared away, the divers had seen a stack of gold and silver bars ten feet wide, six feet high, and forty feet long. On and around the pile of precious metal were heavy gold chains, candelabras, and piles of enormous emeralds. They brought so much to the surface that day that the salvage boat almost sank! It took months to excavate the site, but finally, they got it all. The total value came to about $400 million. Fisher had given everything to find and get that treasure.

Jesus told a couple of stories that closely parallel Mel Fisher's quest. He said, "The kingdom of heaven is like treasure hidden in a field. When a man found it, he hid it again, and then in his joy went and sold all he had and bought that field. Again, the kingdom of heaven is like a merchant looking for fine pearls. When he found one of great value, he went away and sold everything he had and bought it" (Matthew 13:44-46). In the first story, the man wasn't looking for anything. He just happened to see the corner of a box that may have been exposed by a rainstorm. In that day, armies fought over Palestine rather routinely, so people often buried their valuables. The owner of this treasure may have died in the conflict, but this man found it. When he saw what it was, he did some quick math and realized he could buy the property if he sold everything he had. And he did. In the second story, the merchant was always looking for fine pearls. When he saw one of great size and beauty, he, too, did some rapid mental math. He sold everything he had to buy that pearl.

In these stories, the treasure and the pearl represent Jesus. Some of us find him when we're not even looking, and some of us find him because we've searched all our lives for him. Either way, the reasonable response is the same: we value him so much that we "sell all we own" to have him. That's what it means to live in light of the cross: we love God with all our hearts and use things to know him and please him—instead of loving things with all our hearts and using God to get them.

In Psalm 27, David said that he found God to be "delightful" or "beautiful." Do you find God to be delightful and beautiful? Do I? The cross is the measure of God's extravagant and unconditional love for us, his commitment to us, and the power of his purpose for us. A friend of mine once said, "I don't think I'll ever get beyond the cross, and I don't want to. It tells me everything I need to know about God." When we realize how much God loves us and how secure we are as his beloved, adopted children, we become the most humble, and yet the boldest, people on earth. We no longer have to prove ourselves to others. We don't compare ourselves to see where we come out on the pecking order, and we don't have to lie (or "shade the truth a bit") to make ourselves look a little better and others a little worse. We're convinced we're loved, so we love; we know we're accepted, so we accept; we are relieved to be forgiven, so we forgive. The essential nature of Jesus is imparted to us, and we take on his purposes, his compassion, and his strength. Paul said, "Your attitude should be the same as that of Christ Jesus" (Philippians 2:5). As we treasure him more, his life begins to flow out of us. What does it look like? Sometimes, the Spirit of God spontaneously overflows in our attitudes and actions, but more often, we make choices to pick God's way over our old sinful ways. Paul told the Galatians, "But the fruit of the Spirit is love, joy, peace, patience, kindness, goodness, faithfulness, gentleness and self-control. Against such things there is no law. Those who belong to Christ Jesus have crucified the sinful nature with its passions and desires" (Galatians 5:22-24).

How do we treat something we treasure? We think about it, and when our minds aren't focused on something else, we drift back to it again. We can't wait to tell others about its beauty or value. We delight in just being near it, looking at it, and enjoying it. And we protect it at all costs. Does this describe your relationship with God? If not, go back to the cross and peer at the lifeless body hanging there for you. Realize that he went to hell so you don't have to, and he offers you the world—if you're humble enough to say, "I need you."

Obeying out of Gratitude

When we grasp the wonder and power of the cross, our hearts are radically transformed. This change, though, continues to change us from the inside out as long as we dig deeper and deeper into the heart of the gospel of grace. The sacrifice of Jesus, his payment of blood, never gets old. Many years ago, Arabella Hankey wrote the beautiful hymn, "I Love to Tell the Story." The first verse and the chorus say:

"I love to tell the story of unseen things above,

Of Jesus and His glory, of Jesus and His love;

I love to tell the story, because I know 'tis true,

It satisfies my longings as nothing else would do.

Refrain:

I love to tell the story,

'Twill be my theme in glory,

To tell the old, old story

Of Jesus and His love.[27]

Let me offer a few suggestions to keep the old story fresh:

Be ruthlessly realistic about human nature.

As Christians, I'm afraid that our heart's default position isn't gratitude but legalism. We keep drifting back to the hope that we can do enough to earn God's acceptance—and win the applause of those watching us, too. But it's never enough. I could serve faithfully, read my Bible, and give everything I own every moment for a thousand years, but all of it put together could never merit God's grace poured out at the cross. When we read the gospels, we realize that Jesus was in a running battle with the legalistic Pharisees. Their sin of self-righteousness wasn't a small matter. They not only ruined their own relationship with God, but they also poisoned others. Jesus told them bluntly, "You nullify the word of God for the sake of your tradition. You hypocrites! Isaiah was right when he prophesied about you:

"These people honor me with their lips,

but their hearts are far from me.

They worship me in vain;

their teachings are but rules taught by men" (Matthew 15:6-9).

---

27 "I Love to Tell the Story," lyrics by Arabella K. Hankey.

Some may say, "Yes, but I never committed adultery, I never abused drugs, and I never killed anyone. Surely God gives me points for that!" I could say the same thing, but sin goes deeper than that. I'm well aware that my heart is desperately wicked, and any attempts to gain leverage with God by keeping rules are just as nauseating to him as the most obvious sins. As long as we believe we can do something to get God to give us what we want, we keep grace at a distance. But when we, like the tax gatherer in the temple, beat our breasts and feel unworthy even to lift our eyes to heaven because we know we're totally unworthy of God's kindness and forgiveness, our hearts are finally open to the grace of God. Then, Jesus is beautiful . . . a treasure and a delight.

In our church gatherings, we put on a happy face like we're attending a masquerade. We may have fought with our spouse and kids in the car on the way over, but as soon as our feet hit the parking lot, we smile and nod. We say, "Isn't this a wonderful day the Lord has made?" "I'm too blessed to be distressed." "Blessings to you, brother and sister." Don't get me wrong. I'm not against speaking affirming words to one another—as long as they come from our hearts, not to cover up our sins. We don't need to tell everyone how rotten our hearts are. They already have suspicions! When we are brutally honest with God about the depravity of our hearts, we're far more humble, more grateful for the blood of Jesus, and more willing to obey for the right reasons. We stop playing church games to impress each other, and we learn to truly love one another. (We'll look at more on these relationships in the next chapter.)

We can all learn a lot from those who follow the 12 Steps of recovery. They begin this process of repentance with the honest appraisal: "We admit that we are powerless over our addiction, and our lives have become unmanageable." Admitting our need for Christ's forgiveness, love, and power is the first step for all of us if we want our hearts to be transformed, but honesty doesn't end with Step 1. We continue to be honest about our sinful desires, destructive behavior, and compulsive demand to control life every time the Spirit of God whispers in our ears to tell us we're drifting away from grace.

Our old, sinful nature still exists after we become believers. Some preachers say it goes away, but Paul tells us that it not only remains in us, it's getting worse! It never learns, and it never improves. It only gets more rotten as we get older. We shouldn't be surprised when we have lustful desires, bitter thoughts, and speak harmful words. That's still part of our nature, but we aren't helpless victims of our sinful desires. God has given us the Scriptures, the Spirit, the encouragement of friends, and the ability to make better choices. I often reflect on the profound truth in this simple poem:

> *"Two natures beat within my breast.*
> *The one is foul; the other is blessed.*
> *The one I love, the other I hate.*
> *The one I feed will dominate!"*

Connect with God in real prayer.

Too often, we offer only grocery lists to God. It's all about us and our wants, but when our hearts are moved by the substitutionary sacrifice of Jesus on the cross, our prayers change in wonderful ways. We spend far more time telling him how much we appreciate his kindness, and we may spend so much time in praise that we forget to ask for anything. But that's okay because we're sure that a gracious, loving Father already knows everything we need.

When we look at the Psalms, the prayer book of the Scriptures, we see a wide variety of expressions. Sometimes, the writer soars in descriptions of God's majesty and glory, but sometimes, he complains that God has let him down. Every emotion known to man is shared in prayer, from despair to hope, from anger to thankfulness, from fear to wonder. Is this how you and I pray? Do we pour out our hearts to our Heavenly Father, or do we utter bland platitudes we don't really believe, rattle off lists of things we demand, or avoid prayer altogether?

Some Christian traditions put a lot of emphasis on confessing sins. This practice reminds us of our depravity and points us back to the cross. Every time of confession reinforces our dependence on God's grace. Sadly, some of these traditions have lost the beauty and power of this practice in prayer. They just go through the motions, or worse, they think that the practice itself—instead of the blood they need to focus on—absolves them of sin. I'm a big fan of *The Godfather* series. Have you ever thought about how many times the crime family committed atrocities while family members were in church for confessions and baptisms? Clearly, the practice had lost its meaning for them. When we use it properly, however, confessing our sins isn't morbid or superficial. It restores the joy of our salvation and inspires us to follow Jesus more closely than ever. The Greek term translated "confession" is *homo logos*. It means to think the same way. When we confess our sins, we think the same way God thinks about our sins, about his forgiveness, and about his purpose for us to live in a way that brings him glory.

As we understand the nature of our relationship with God—adoption through propitiation—two things happen at once: we trust him more because he's proven his love, and we are far more honest with him about everything in our lives. And when we're honest with God, he delights in us.

Find partners in faith.

God intended the Christian life to be a team sport. We need each other, and in fact, we may learn a lot of facts on our own, but we won't truly grow unless we're in community with other believers. We can, however, lose ourselves in a church or organization of more than a few dozen people. We need to find a few, maybe two or three, who become our partners in running the race with Jesus. Paul had Barnabas, then Silas, and then Timothy. Susan and I each have friends who love us enough to speak the truth to us. A group of men has made a commitment to talk to each other regularly, and after sharing what's going on in their lives, they ask three questions:

- What have you struggled with most in your life since we last talked?
- Where have you seen God at work most powerfully?
- What haven't you told me that you need to tell me?

These questions help these men take off their masks and speak the truth to one another. They began with a heartfelt commitment to honesty, and these questions take them a step farther each time they talk.

Serve humbly and gladly.

When there was no servant to wash dusty feet before the Last Supper, Jesus took the role of the lowest servant to perform that task. Like most of us, the disciples were more interested in competing with each other for power and fame, but Jesus modeled a different way to live. After he finished, he told them, "Do you understand what I have done for you? You call me 'Teacher' and 'Lord,' and rightly so, for that is what I am. Now that I, your Lord and Teacher, have washed your feet, you also should wash one another's feet. I have set you an example that you should do as I have done for you. I tell you the truth, no servant is greater than his master, nor is a messenger greater than the one who sent him. Now that you know these things, you will be blessed if you do them" (John 13:12-17).

Our humility is fueled by a genuine passion to please our Father. Because we've been set free from the bondage of sin, we want others to experience the same freedom, joy, and purpose. Before Auca Indians in Ecuador martyred him, Jim Elliot wrote in this journal, "He makes His ministers a flame of fire. Am I ignitable? God deliver me from the dread asbestos of 'other things.' Saturate me with the oil of the Spirit that I may be aflame. But flame is transient, often short lived. Canst thou bear this, my soul-short life? Make me thy fuel, Flame of God." Each of the eleven remaining disciples suffered and died for the cause of Christ. Because they were overwhelmed with the death of Jesus for them, nothing mattered but to love him in return and give everything they had for him.

Our acts of service can be as simple as speaking a kind word to a hurting person or as structured as establishing an organization to care for people. The list of options is endless, but it all starts with a desire to make a difference in the lives of others because Jesus has made a difference in our lives.

Become a student of truth.

Spiritual insight doesn't happen by magic, and it doesn't occur by osmosis. We gain perception from diving deeply into the truth of God's word and trusting the Spirit to illumine his truth to our hearts. Study takes effort, but it's well worth it. Like learning to play the violin, learning to study the Bible begins with a steep curve, but after a while, the benefits are remarkable. Paul wrote Timothy about the value of knowing the Scriptures: "But as for you, continue in what you have learned and have become convinced of, because you know those from whom you learned it, and how from infancy you have known the holy Scriptures, which are able to make you wise for salvation through faith in Christ Jesus. All Scripture is God-breathed and is useful for teaching, rebuking, correcting and training in righteousness, so that the man of God may be thoroughly equipped for every good work" (2 Timothy 3:14-17).

I believe that a person's spiritual growth is dependent upon and a reflection of the study of God's word. We simply won't grow beyond our grasp of biblical truth. Is it worth the effort? Yes, indeed. The more we explore the truths about God's greatness and grace, the more he inspires us to love him, equips us to handle difficulties, and directs us to relate to people at home, at work, and in church with love and strength. Three millennia ago, David wrote, "Your word is a lamp to my feet and a light for my path" (Psalm 119:105). It still is.

Develop discipline.

God never promised that following Jesus would be easy. In our affluent culture, the expectation of a life of plenty has crept into the hearts of countless Christians, leaving them spiritually weak and vulnerable to the enemy's deceptions. Sometimes, I hear people talk about sacrifice, but some of them don't really understand what it's about. An alcoholic says he gave up drinking for Jesus, an adulterer stops having illicit sex and becomes a faithful spouse "for Christ," or a compulsive shopper says she cut up her credit cards for God. No, they gave those things up because those behaviors were destroying their lives. True sacrifice is giving up things that we deemed as valuable, but we've concluded that Christ is worth far more. Paul was the Top Gun in his world of theology and leadership, but he said he counted it all as rubbish because of "the surpassing value of knowing Christ" (Philippians 3:7-10).

The cross is the dividing line of motivation. On one side, we love power, prestige, and possessions, and we use God to get them. On the other, we are blown away by the love of God plainly demonstrated in the shed blood of Jesus, and we're willing to do anything—anything!—to please him. Discipline, then, isn't just gutting out some hard choices. It's going back to the reason we make choices. The more we focus on Christ's sacrifice for us, the more we're willing and thrilled to sacrifice for him. C. T. Studd was the most famous athlete in England in the latter part of the 19th century, but he answered God's call to go to Africa to tell people about Jesus. Did he regret living in poverty and loneliness instead of wealth and public acclaim? Not at all. His choices were shaped and fueled by his grasp of the cross. He said, "If Jesus Christ be God and died for me, then no sacrifice can be too great for me to make for him."

Authenticity

There is no Christianity apart from the cross, and there is no spiritual vitality for believers without a strong grasp of Calvary. The blood of Jesus is the beginning of our salvation, the middle of our growth, and the ultimate promise of glory forever. Other religions articulate principles to tell people how to live. They have a measure of wisdom and insight about people and relationships, but Christianity is categorically different. Our leader wasn't just a wise man—he gave himself to pay the price none of us could ever pay. When we are thoroughly convinced that we're forgiven, we realize we don't have to wear a mask any longer to hide our shame. An understanding of the cross inevitably leads to an authentic life of peace, love, and joyful obedience to our Father.

Let me ask you a few questions: Has the Lord whispered to your heart as you've read this chapter? Perhaps he has reinforced your thankfulness that Christ has paid the price for you, and you're his beloved, adopted child. But maybe as you've read these pages, you realize your heart is cold toward God. You've tried as hard as you can to win his acceptance, but it's never been enough to fill the hole in your heart. A rich, life-changing relationship with God isn't earned by trying harder. We can only enter this relationship by a single door: the one opened when Jesus paid the entry fee in full. Or maybe you gave up trying a long time ago and resent God (and anyone else) who has the audacity to talk about the power of the blood of Jesus to rescue us from sin and death.

As God's child, are you loyal to him, devoted to his cause, and thrilled to see him use you to touch people's lives?

Is confession of sin a burden or a pathway to a richer relationship with God? Are you realistic about the existence of two natures in your soul, or are you surprised when you sin?

Do you see Jesus as your most valuable treasure? Do you delight in him? Are you happy to make the reasonable choice to forsake everything to know him better?

Propitiation is a strange word to most of us, but the concept speaks loudly and clearly about the extent God was willing to go for us. As a loving parent, he gave his life for us. Remembering his sacrifice, and studying it so that it seeps into the nooks and crannies of our souls, enables us to live as his children in humility and gratitude in the shadow of the cross.

Reflect on Garfield T. Haywood's powerful hymn, "I See a Crimson Stream":

"On Cal'vry's hill of sorrow

Where sin's demands were paid,

And rays of hope for tomorrow
Across our path were laid.

Refrain:
I see a crimson stream of blood,
It flows from Calvary,
Its waves which reach the throne of God,
Are sweeping over me.

Today no condemnation
Abides to turn away
My soul from His salvation,
He's in my heart to stay.

When gloom and sadness whisper,
"You've sinned—no use to pray,"
I look away to Jesus,
And He tells me to say:

And when we reach the portal
Where life forever reigns,
The ransomed hosts' grand final
Will be this glad refrain."[28]

---

28 "I See a Crimson Stream," Garfield T. Haywood, 1920.

Think about it...

1. Describe the importance of Dr. Packer's definition of the Christian faith: "adoption through propitiation."

2. How is being adopted by God different from seeing Christianity as a set of rules to follow? How does adoption affect our love for God and our willingness to obey him?

3. How do you treat the most valuable thing you own? How do you treat Jesus? What are the similarities and differences?

4. What are some reasons we're afraid to take off our masks in church? Who are some honest, genuine people who don't play games to impress people? Are their lives attractive to you? Why or why not?

5. Which of the practices mentioned in this chapter—confession, accountability, service, and Bible study—is an area that needs your attention? How will a growing proficiency help you walk more closely with Jesus?

6. Look at the questions at the end of the chapter. Which of them is the most challenging to you? Which is the most inspiring? Explain your answer.

Breaking Down Barriers

" Our life is full of brokenness—broken relationships, bro-

ken promises, broken expectations. How can we live with

that brokenness without becoming bitter and resentful

except by returning again and again to God's faithful

presence in our lives?"

—Henri Nouwen

After Judas left the last dinner to betray Jesus to the Jewish authorities, Jesus turned to his followers and told them, "A new
command I give you: Love one another. As I have loved you, so you
must love one another. By this all men will know that you are my
disciples, if you love one another" (John 13:34-35). In those last
hours, Jesus' thinking was crystallized by the terrible reality of the
suffering he faced the next day. Like a prisoner on death row making
his last walk, he focused only on the things that were of paramount
importance. One of the things he talked about was unity in the body
of Christ. He told them to love each other. How? In the same way he
loved them. How much? To the extent he loved them.

Bridges or Barriers?

After Jesus and the remaining disciples left the Upper Room, they walked to a garden. There, Jesus poured out his heart to the Father. He prayed for the eleven men who would carry the message of his sacrifice of blood to the world, and then he said, "My prayer is not for them alone. I pray also for those who will believe in me through their message, that all of them may be one, Father, just as you are in me and I am in you. May they also be in us so that the world may believe that you have sent me. I have given them the glory that you gave me, that they may be one as we are one: I in them and you in me. May they be brought to complete unity to let the world know that you sent me and have loved them even as you have loved me" (John 17:20-23).

Church history has been marked by some wonderful stories of believers sacrificing themselves for each other. In famine, war, natural disasters, accidents, and all kinds of life and death struggles, some Christians saw others "as more important than themselves." They were willing to give, love, and die for one another with no strings attached. But far too often, Christians fail miserably to answer Jesus' call to love sacrificially and build bridges of unity. We argue about petty things, get our feelings hurt at the drop of a hat, compete with each other for applause, thirst for power over each other, and compare everything from hats to houses so we can feel we're a little bit better than others. Sadly, instead of bridges, we've built barriers.

We like to think of the early church as the Golden Age. Fifty days after the resurrection, God chose another feast, Pentecost, to send his Spirit to invade the lives of believers. It was a glorious day, and in the weeks that followed, it radically changed the nature of individuals and relationships. We get a glimpse of what Jesus was talking about when he prayed for unity when Luke tells us about the way believers loved each other in Jerusalem in those early days: "They devoted themselves to the apostles' teaching and to the fellowship, to the breaking of bread and to prayer. Everyone was filled with awe, and many wonders and miraculous signs were done by the apostles. All the believers were together and had everything in common. Selling their possessions and goods, they gave to anyone as he had need. Every day they continued to meet together in the temple courts. They broke bread in their homes and ate together with glad and sincere hearts, praising God and enjoying the favor of all the people. And the Lord added to their number daily those who were being saved" (Acts 2:42-47).

Unfortunately, we don't read about this kind of unity happening very often in the rest of Acts and the letters of the New Testament. Even as Christians—bought by the blood of Christ and sealed by his Spirit for a life of love and purpose—our default mode is selfishness. When Paul wrote to the church in Galatia, he needed to correct their theology and their behavior. They had forgotten that the sacrifice of Jesus freed them from the requirements and penalty of the law. They had drifted back to keeping rules to prove they were acceptable to God. Paul's letter was fierce! Near the end, he addressed the natural result of forgetting grace: resentment, comparison, and division. He explained that grace is the only sure foundation for loving one another. In the church, we must guard against "spiritual autoimmune disease," in which spiritual white cells see normal cells within the body as enemies and try to destroy them. Paul wrote, "You, my brothers, were called to be free. But do not use your freedom to indulge the sinful nature; rather, serve one another in love. The entire law is summed up in a single command: 'Love your neighbor as yourself.' If you keep on biting and devouring each other, watch out or you will be destroyed by each other" (Galatians 5:13-15).

Is it possible for a human body to "bite and devour" healthy cells, destroying life? Absolutely. As we saw earlier in this book, sometimes white blood cells mistakenly attack healthy cells in the blood, causing disastrous results. The immune system fails to recognize components of the body as normal. It then creates *autoantibodies* that attack its own cells, tissues, or organs. This causes inflammation and damage, and it leads to autoimmune disorders. For example, *autoimmune hemolytic anemia* is a group of disorders that attack red blood cells as if they were substances foreign to the body. Like other cases of anemia, the person may experience shortness of breath, tiredness, and jaundice. When the destruction of healthy red cells persists for a long period of time, the spleen may enlarge, resulting in a sense of abdominal fullness and pain.

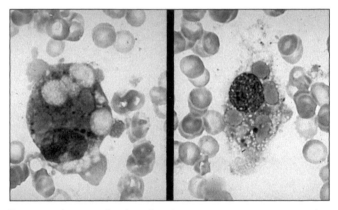

Figure 12. An example of erythrophagocytosis, an autoimmune phenomenon in which red cells are ingested by white cells.

God intends for his body to be healthy, nourish each other, protect each other, and carry harmful waste away. He grieves when his people exemplify an autoimmune disorder by biting and devouring each other. Jesus said the gates of hell can't prevail against the church.

This means that Satan can't defeat the church, but we can bite and devour each other. We're our own worst enemy.

In the Beginning and From the Top

All blood cells in our bodies come from a single source: *pluripotent*, or *hematopoietic stem cells* (HSCs), which are formed in the bone marrow and contain cells with long-term and short-term regeneration capacities. Each of the types of cells in our blood has different structures and functions, but they all are created at the same source. Each of the billions of cells in the bloodstream of a human body has a unique role, but they share the same DNA.

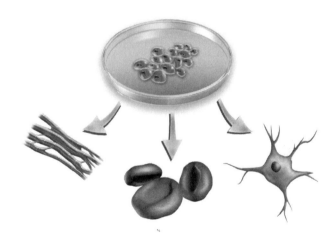

Figure 13. Differentiating hematopoietic stem cells.

God has orchestrated the human body to create and place the right cells in the right places at the right times to keep us healthy. In the same way, the body of Christ is made up of billions of Christians who are diverse in their ethnicity, cultural backgrounds, talents, and abilities, but each one was "birthed" at the single source of spiritual life, the HSC of Christ's blood. God sovereignly places each of us in the community of faith, the bloodstream of corporate spiritual life, so we can play our unique roles to keep the body of Christ strong and healthy.

In the study of the function of B and T lymphocytes in AIDS patients, doctors realized that the body was overwhelmed with the virus when the number of T cells fell below a critical level. This led to the discovery that the body has the ability to regulate the production of various cells, and even to redirect fully mature, functioning cells, such as B cells, to mutate and become a different type of cell, T cells. In the body of Christ, the Lord gives us the ability to adapt to the changing needs in our environment so that we take advantage of opportunities to expand the kingdom, teach truth to counter the destructive force of deception, and heal the hurts of wounded people. Jesus Christ is our HSC, the hematopoietic stem cell from which all of us originate. When we're born again, the Spirit inserts his spiritual DNA, the nature of Christ, into us, forming us into particular "cells" in his body, mutating us when needs arise, and using us to nurture, protect, and heal his body. We may be black or white, Chinese or Indian, Pentecostal or Baptist, rich or poor, expressive in praise or reflective, worshipping in mega-churches or in storefronts—but we all are formed from a single source to accomplish his purposes. We are very different, but with a common purpose; our differences result in greater unity, not division. In the interworking of cells in our blood, each type performs various functions in very different ways, but we'll die if each cell doesn't fulfill its purpose. In the same way, we need to learn to appreciate—instead of despise—the contributions of each person in the body of Christ—even those who are far different from us. In America and the western world, we value independence at all costs, but the biblical value of interdependence is higher, stronger, and more important.

To illustrate the intricate and powerful interdependence of Christians, Paul used the now familiar analogy of the human body. In some diseases and disorders, the nerves of parts of the body aren't adequately connected to the head, and the person's limbs jerk uncontrollably. To function properly, each part must be intimately connected to the brain. In the body of Christ, the principle is the same. We won't be able to walk, talk, or chew gum spiritually if we aren't taking our orders from our head, Jesus Christ. To illustrate this point, Paul wrote the Ephesians, "Speaking the truth in love, we will in all things grow up into him who is the Head, that is, Christ. From him the whole body, joined and held together by every supporting ligament, grows and builds itself up in love, as each part does its work" (Ephesians 4:15-16). And he explained to the Christians in Corinth that every person, no matter how obscure, is vital to the proper functioning of Christ's body. He told them, "Now the body is not made up of one part but of many. . . . But in fact God has arranged the parts in the body, every one of them, just as he wanted them to be. If they were all one part, where would the body be? As it is, there are many parts, but one body" (1 Corinthians 12:14, 18-20).

However, Paul was under no illusions that believers were going to usher in the ideal in human relationships. Like every other advance in our spiritual lives, each step would be a fight. The battle lines were clearly drawn in the early church. For the first few years, virtually all believers were Jews. When Peter and Paul went to the Gentiles and they trusted Christ as their savior, a crisis occurred. The animosity between these two races and cultures threatened to destroy the young body of Christ. A council in Jerusalem debated the issue and finally settled the theological fact: Jesus came for all people, Jews and Gentiles alike. The implementation of this truth, though, needed much more than a signed document. Everywhere Paul traveled, he had to teach people what Jesus meant by "loving one another as I have loved you." Old hatreds died hard, and only a deep understanding and true experience of the love of God through the blood of Jesus overcome them. When he wrote to the Christians in the port city of Ephesus, he recognized that they were Gentiles who traditionally hated the Jews. He didn't put a Band Aid over their preconceptions; instead, he gave them a transfusion. He wrote, "Therefore, remember that formerly you who are Gentiles by birth and called 'uncircumcised' by those who call themselves 'the circumcision' (that done in the body by the hands of men)—remember that at that time you were separate from Christ, excluded from citizenship in Israel and foreigners to the covenants of the promise, without hope and without God in the world. But now in Christ Jesus you who once were far away have been brought near through the blood of Christ" (Ephesians 2:11-13).

For most of us, the conflicts and psychological distance we experience with other believers aren't as deep and dramatic as the cultural rift between Jews and Gentiles. Of course, there are ethnic and cultural differences between people of different colors and socioeconomic backgrounds, but most of our divisions come from differing preferences, misunderstandings, and unresolved hurt feelings—things that could be easily remedied by a little conversation, a touch of kindness, and a dose of forgiveness. When we allow little hurts to remain unhealed for a long time, the infection of resentment and distrust festers into major problems that require much more effort to heal—if, indeed, we ever address them.

To the Ephesians, Paul said that the only hope for unity in the body of Christ was the blood of Jesus. But the blood of Christ wasn't just a nice theological doctrine to be dusted off from time to time. It had (and still has) the power to transform hearts, and then to revolutionize relationships. When we truly embrace the grace of Christ, we forgive past hurts, reach out to understand, and provide our resources to care for those we previously despised. In graphic language, Paul explained how Christ achieves unity among us: "For he himself is our peace, who has made the two one and has destroyed the barrier, the dividing wall of hostility, by abolishing in his flesh the law with its commandments and regulations. His purpose was to create in himself one new man out of the two, thus making peace, and in this one body to reconcile both of them to God through the cross, by which he put to death their hostility. He came and preached peace to you who were far away and peace to those who were near. For through him we both have access to the Father by one Spirit" (Ephesians 2:14-18).

Jesus didn't stand back wringing his hands pleading, "Won't you try to get along?" He made peace the hard way, by "putting to death the hostility" and making sure people in conflict find common ground through his blood. In medicine, we talk often about a patient "fighting" a disease. The term applies in the spiritual world as well. A friend who is a psychologist told me that we have to "grab our selfish nature by the throat and strangle it because it won't die quietly." Jesus put our hostility to death at the cross, and we have to fight to put it to death in our hearts every day. It's much easier to "learn church" than to "learn Christ." One only requires that we figure out how to play the game so we look spiritual and holy, but the other forces us to be ruthlessly honest about the sin that blackens our hearts and poisons our relationships, and then experience and express Christ's forgiveness.

We don't enjoy unity when we focus on unity. We only find true unity in the body of Christ when we turn our eyes off ourselves and our relationships and put them on the cross, the source of forgiveness, love, and compassion. We can't give away something we don't possess, and I'm afraid that the poverty of love for others in families and the church is a reflection of the emptiness in our hearts. We will only love others to the extent that we experience the love of God (1 John 4:10-11); we'll only forgive others to the degree that we are convinced we've been forgiven (Colossians 3:13); and we'll only accept others if we're thrilled that God has accepted us (Romans 15:7). All of these are directly connected to our grasp of the power and the beauty of the cross.

Reach Out to the Unlovely

How can we tell if the love of Jesus has penetrated the tough shell of our hearts? There are many ways to see if our faith is genuine, but surely one of them is our willingness to love the unlovely. Jesus said that when his love permeates our hearts, we see people in a different way. We don't think of them as beautiful or ugly, rich or poor, or contributing to our happiness or detracting from it. We see them as people for whom Christ died. No matter what their circumstances in life, they are more valuable to God than all the wealth on the planet. If we see them through his eyes, we'll value them, too. Someday, every person on earth will stand before God to give an account for his or her life. If we see people through the lens of eternity, each one takes on inestimable value. In his famous sermon, "The Weight of Glory," C. S. Lewis observed that an eternal perspective shows us there are "no ordinary people." He said, "It is a serious thing to live in a society of possible gods and goddesses, to remember that the dullest and most uninteresting person you talk to may one day be a creature which, if you saw it now, you would be strongly tempted to worship, or else a horror and a corruption such as you now meet, if at all, only in a nightmare. All day long we are, in some degree, helping each other to one or other of these destinations. It is in the light of these overwhelming possibilities, it is with the awe and the circumspection proper to them, that we should conduct all our dealings with one another, all friendships, all loves, all play, all politics. There are no *ordinary* people. You have never talked to a mere mortal."[29]

One man admitted that he's always had a hard time even being cordial to ugly people. When Jesus changed his heart, he made a decision to look unlovely people in the eye and speak to them. He had always looked *past* them, but now he looked *at* them. He said that this discipline had given him a love for them he had never had before, and God has used him to share his kindness to people who desperately need an act of love—even a small act like looking into their eyes.

Some people aren't just unlovely; they're nasty! Even then, the blood of Jesus changes our hearts and gives us the ability to love them—not to condone their behavior, but to love them in spite of it. Jesus told the crowds, "You have heard that it was said, 'Love your neighbor and hate your enemy.' But I tell you: Love your enemies and pray for those who persecute you, that you may be sons of your Father in heaven. He causes his sun to rise on the evil and the good, and sends rain on the righteous and the unrighteous. If you love those who love you, what reward will you get? Are not even the tax collectors doing that?" (Matthew 5:43-46) If the sacrifice of Christ is

---

29 C. S. Lewis, "The Weight of Glory," a message delivered at the Church of St. Mary the Virgin, Oxford, June 8, 1942, online at www.verber.com/mark/xian/weight-of-glory.pdf.

real to us, one of the most striking signs is that we love, forgive, and accept people who have been our enemies.

Speak Words of Kindness

In our culture, we laugh at sin on sit-coms every night, and we use sarcasm to communicate with people all day, every day. We may think these forms of language don't have much impact, but they do. Our words have the capacity to heal or destroy. We need to take a good, long look at the words we use in our homes, our work, our neighborhoods, and in church.

A kind or affirming word spoken with sincerity can change the world—or at least a few days—for the person receiving it. A friend of mine received a nice compliment, and he told me, "I'll live on that for a week!" We're starved for simple words that say, "I love you," "You're important to me," "I believe in you," "You're really talented." These and a thousand variations impart life to the people in our lives. To create space for words like these (in our hearts and in our mouths), we need to stop saying things that act as a corrosive agent to eat away the other person's sense of security. Why do we use harmful words? Because they are effective in controlling people. Our goal, though, is love, not control. Paul wrote, "Do not let any un-wholesome talk come out of your mouths, but only what is helpful for building others up according to their needs, that it may benefit those who listen. And do not grieve the Holy Spirit of God, with whom you were sealed for the day of redemption" (Ephesians 4:29-30). Hateful, condemning, sarcastic words grieve God and crush the spirit of those we're talking to.

Where do we find affirming words to say? Jesus told us, "Each tree is recognized by its own fruit. People do not pick figs from thornbushes, or grapes from briers. The good man brings good things out of the good stored up in his heart, and the evil man brings evil things out of the evil stored up in his heart. For out of the overflow of his heart his mouth speaks" (Luke 6:44-45). Again, we need to look into our hearts to see the source of our words. When we go back to the cross, we realize we are deeply loved, completely forgiven, and fully accepted by the grace of God. We don't have to compete with anyone any longer to prove ourselves, and we don't have to use angry words to control people. When the love of God overflows from our hearts, we speak loving, affirming, positive (and sometimes, appropriately corrective) words to the people around us.

Take Action

In some families, and sometimes in the family of God, gracious words are disconnected from gracious actions. When people don't see consistency and continuity, they have every reason to wonder if our words mean anything at all. As the old saying goes, "It's not enough just to talk the talk; we have to also walk the walk." In the opening chapters of Acts, people gave all they had to provide for people in need. They understood that everything they owned was God's, and they gladly put their resources at his disposal. The willingness to give comes from the heartfelt conviction that God's kingdom is more important than our comfort. In Paul's second letter to the Corinthians, he reported that the church in Macedonia had this perspective. He wrote, "For I testify that they gave as much as they were able, and even beyond their ability. Entirely on their own, they urgently pleaded with us for the privilege of sharing in this service to the saints. And they did not do as we expected, but they gave themselves first to the Lord and then to us in keeping with God's will" (2 Corinthians 8:3-5). Paul didn't have to twist their arms to make them give—they gave willingly, generously, and even hilariously, because they realized they were primarily giving to God. We may be able to fake our love by hugging people and uttering spiritual platitudes, but writing a check shows what's really in our hearts.

To illustrate the importance of showing our love by sacrificial action, Jesus told a parable. He was talking with the religious leaders that hated a group of people known as Samaritans. They were biracial, descendents of Jews who intermarried with Gentiles after one of the foreign invasions and captivities. The Jews saw themselves as God's chosen race, and indeed they were, but God's plan wasn't to turn them into a holy huddle. He wanted them to carry the message of grace to every person on earth. They failed miserably. Instead, the Jews couldn't even get along with their closest neighbors, people who had a large share of Jewish blood coursing through their veins.

In his conversation with the religious leaders, one of them asked Jesus how he could have eternal life. Jesus said to love God with your heart, soul and mind, and love your neighbor as yourself. The man, though, wanted to be sure Jesus meant his *Jewish* neighbors, not any Samaritans or other Gentiles. In response, Jesus turned his world upside down. His story told about a Jewish man who was robbed and beaten, left for dead on the side of the road. A priest came by and saw the broken and bleeding man, but he didn't stop to help. Then a Levite came by. He, too, gave only a glance and kept going. Then, a Samaritan came along the road. His heart broke when he saw the Jewish man lying in the gutter. He bandaged his wounds, put him on his donkey, and took him to an inn to recover. Before he left, the Samaritan gave the innkeeper enough money to feed and house the man for two weeks, offering to pay any extra when he came back. It was an astounding act of kindness, but what struck those listening was the point that the one who showed the love of God wasn't the one they expected—it was the one they hated, a Samaritan. He was the true neighbor to the man who had been robbed and beaten.

Who are the people we pass by each day in our offices and neighborhoods? Their wounds may not be physical. They may be emotionally broken and spiritually bleeding. They may exhibit their hurts in withdrawal or in outbursts of rage. They need someone to step into their lives to bandage their hurts and stay connected to them during the healing process. Too often, we see someone in need and mumble, "I'll pray for you." We may utter a quick prayer, but we really don't want to be bothered by the other person's distress. We want our lives to remain uncluttered and squeaky clean. If we look at the life of Jesus, his life was one of sacrificial service, always reaching out to touch lepers, the blind, the lame, the sick, prostitutes, tax gatherers, and outcasts of every kind. When we say we want to be more like Jesus, that's what it means. We treat others the way we want to be treated. The golden rule is still the measuring stick of active love.

Pay It Forward

Acts of sacrificial service can change the culture of a family, a church, a business, or any other organization. During World War II, the Japanese used 180,000 Asian laborers and 60,000 Allied prisoners of war to build a railroad through the jungle from Bangkok, Thailand, to Rangoon, Burma (now Myanmar). It wasn't called "The Death Railway" for nothing. The conditions were so brutal that over 400 men died for every mile of track built, about 106,000 in all. With little food, brutal beatings, and death in the air each day, the men soon lived like animals. They despised those who got a morsel of food more than they received, and they hated those who didn't have to work quite as hard. The esprit de corps of the Allied armies deteriorated into barbarism.

At the end of one day's hard work, the Japanese captain ordered all the prisoners to come back and stand at attention. He announced that a shovel was missing when his soldiers counted them after work had stopped that day. He held up a pistol and said that if the thief didn't confess, he would begin shooting prisoners. They knew this was no idle threat. Suddenly, a voice was heard from the back of the formation: "I did it. I took the shovel." A haggard man stepped forward to face the captain. In an instant, the captain picked up a shovel and beat him to death in front of his comrades.

A few minutes later, a second count showed that the shovel hadn't been missing after all. The man had sacrificed himself to save other men, and they all realized the meaning of what he had done. Suddenly, the atmosphere of the camp changed. Men who had been at each other's throats the day before now understood they had another shot at life, a gift from one of their friends. They stopped hating each other and began looking for ways to help each other. When one of them was sick, the others picked up the slack. They freely gave support, food, and love to one another—all because one man had died for the rest.

The death of Christ on the cross affects us as a community as well as individually. As Americans, we may be rugged individualists, but that's not how God wants us to live. When we grasp Christ's sacrifice of blood, we're willing to sacrifice our time, our money, and our hearts for those around us. And as we make even small sacrifices, the people who receive our love "pay it forward" to love others. It's a beautiful thing to see. Hatred is contagious in close quarters, but so is compassion—and we don't need antibodies for love.

Be a Minister of Reconciliation

You don't have to be a counselor or pastor to know that most people carry deep hurts and unresolved anger with them every day. Wounded people may try to suppress their pain, but it spills out in all kinds of ways. As the title of a book informs us, hurt people hurt people. As people who have been set free from the bondage of bitterness, we have the privilege of being ministers of reconciliation in the lives of hurting people around us. Everyone needs to be reconciled to God, and many people around us need God to use us to help them mend broken relationships—or if the other party isn't willing to take steps of reconciliation, each of us can, "so far as it depends on [us], be at peace with all men" (Romans 12:18).

Jesus commanded us to love others "just as I have loved you." We don't have to guess what love looks like. We only need to see how Jesus loved people. He taught about love, but he didn't leave it there. He demonstrated his love in countless ways to innumerable people. He even loved his enemies so much that he died for them, too. Nothing could stop him. His love, though, was never sentimental. He was honest about the sin he saw in people's lives, and he called them out. It's not love to excuse an addict's lies, a teenager's rebellion, or a spouse's porn habits. We love "in deed and truth" when we speak the reality of a situation, call people to repentance, and offer the possibility to reconcile broken relationships and rebuild trust. We are foolish to trust untrustworthy people, but love opens the door to see if they'll come back in and do the hard work to earn our trust again. God commands us to forgive, but he never commands us to trust people who haven't proven to be trustworthy.

When we walk past friends and family members who are ruining their lives, we aren't showing them Christ's love. We can't make people change, but we can hold a mirror up and let them see the damage they're causing. Paul told the Galatians, "Brothers, if someone is caught in a sin, you who are spiritual should restore him gently" (Galatians 6:1). And he told the Christians in Thessalonica to get involved in people's lives by tailoring their approach to their needs. He said, "And we urge you, brothers, warn those who are idle, encourage the timid, help the weak, be patient with everyone. Make sure that nobody pays back wrong for wrong, but always try to be kind to each other and to everyone else" (1 Thessalonians 5:14-15).

We can be ministers of reconciliation—mending relationships with God and with others—when we have the courage and develop the skill to step into people's lives at the point of their need and speak words of grace and truth to them. The process of healing, restoring relationships, and rebuilding trust requires another step: our consistent presence to help them navigate these rough waters. When we help people in this way, we certainly need to be realistic. Even if we give them true wisdom and great advice, we need to realize they are facing life's most difficult challenge, and many will bail out. The most courageous people on earth are the ones who are willing to face their inner demons and family adversaries. I have the utmost respect for them—and for those who help them. Englishman Edmund Burke accurately observed, "The only thing necessary for the triumph of evil is for good men to do nothing." Let's not allow the triumph of evil in the lives of those around us. It's not enough to notice evil. We have to get under the rock with people and help them overcome it. It's much easier to stay in our comfort zones and avoid helping people in sticky situations, but when we extend a hand to help them, we are loving people like Jesus loves them.

A Shrinking World

Only a century ago, people took weeks or months to sail to distant lands to do business, see their families, or take the gospel to places where it had not been heard. Today, a few hours on a plane gets us there. In the past few years, the Internet has built a web of connections around the world that was unimaginable only a short time ago. One man said that he understood how closely the world was connected when he, an American, was in Peru shopping at a store owned and run by a Vietnamese family. "We're all in this together now," he remarked.

As global citizens, we need old fault lines of differences to continue to be torn down by the cross. Increasing global proximity can produce either conflict or compassion, and we must choose compassion. We have opportunities to show God's love to refugees in Darfur, dig wells for people with dirty water in India, and provide school supplies and food for a child in Chile. The sacrifice of Christ is relevant in Judea, Samaria, and the remotest parts of the earth, not only in our own Jerusalems. The Christian faith is not an American possession. In fact, there are parts of the world where the gospel is spreading faster than here in the United States. Soon, China will have more Christians than the entire population of our country. Many people around the world have far fewer consumer goods than we possess, but they love God with all their hearts. In some parts of the world, people despise us and say we're soft because they don't see any willingness to sacrifice for the cause we say we believe in. Far too often, they're absolutely right. We're "third soil people." The freshness of the gospel has been choked out by "the worries of the world and the deceitfulness of riches." We need to wake up to what's really important.

Jesus said, "To whom much is given, much is required" (Luke 12:48). Instead of getting caught up in the rat race for more, faster, and higher, we'll do well to stop, think, and learn to use the incredible resources God has given us to advance his kingdom rather than spend them primarily on our pleasure and comfort. Not long ago, I preached at a church in Liberia. When I finished, they asked me to preach again—right then. They had been standing for hours, but they were so hungry for God that they wanted to hear the word even more. The conditions at the church were primitive. The building had only one light bulb, so we had to finish before the sun went down. They had no running water, and little sanitation, but they didn't care. They love God and want to follow him with all their hearts. In most of our churches, pastors get dirty looks and critical emails if the service goes ten minutes longer than the scheduled time to finish. We may have material wealth, but we have a lot to learn from our brothers and sisters around the world about loving the Lord with all our hearts and our neighbors as ourselves.

The opportunities to share the love of God are almost endless. When we have a global consciousness, we care about people who are very different than us. We learn to look past skin color, hygiene, housing, strange customs, and everything else that might have caused us to withdraw into the safe cocoons of our own world. We have the opportunity to touch lives around the planet—if we'll only see every potential interaction as a way to be the feet, hands, and voice of Jesus to them.

When Charles Wesley came to Christ, he was so overwhelmed with the grace of God poured out on him by the blood of Jesus that he sat down to write a hymn of praise. The words that came to him that night are sung with passion and humility by groups of people who want to praise God together for his grace. Wesley wrote:

"Where shall my wondering soul begin?
How shall I all to heaven aspire?
A slave redeemed from death and sin,
A brand plucked from eternal fire,
How shall I equal triumphs raise,
Or sing my great Deliverer's praise?

O how shall I the goodness tell,
Father, which Thou to me hast showed?
That I, a child of wrath and hell,
I should be called a child of God,
Should know, should feel my sins forgiven,
Blessed with this antepast of Heaven!

Outcasts of men, to you I call,
Harlots, and publicans, and thieves!
He spreads His arms to embrace you all;
Sinners alone His grace receives;
No need of Him the righteous have;
He came the lost to seek and save.

Come, O my guilty brethren, come,
Groaning beneath your load of sin,
His bleeding heart shall make you room,
His open side shall take you in;
He calls you now, invites you home;

Come, O my guilty brethren, come!

For you the purple current flowed

In pardons from His wounded side,

Languished for you the eternal God,

For you the Prince of glory died:

Believe, and all your sins forgiven;

Only believe, and yours is Heaven!"[30]

All those who have been bought by the blood of Jesus gladly sing this song together, and their differences evaporate in their praise. The cross revolutionizes relationships. If we live in the default mode of legalism and rule keeping, we'll compete with each other so we can feel superior to people around us. And if we devote our lives to the pursuit of pleasure, we won't care about others at all. We'll be completely consumed with having all we want right now. But the gospel of Christ transforms us. The blood of Jesus heals our broken hearts, nourishes our souls, and overflows into the lives of others. Because we've experienced his wonderful grace, we make choices to love the unlovely, make sacrifices for those who can't pay us back, change our language to speak words of kindness, change our lifestyles to reflect God's values, and pay his love forward to everyone we meet. That kind of love changes the world.

---

30 "Where Shall My Wondering Soul Begin?", lyrics by Charles Wesley, 1739, music by Dmitri S. Bortniansky, 1825.

Think about it...

1. How have you seen Christians "bite and devour one another"? How did it affect them? How did it affect you?

2. When and how have you seen Christ's prayer for unity among believers answered? What impact did it have on people?

3. What difference does it make to understand that all of us come from the same spiritual source, just like all types of cells in the blood all come from HSCs?

4. What are some choices people (like you) can make to love, forgive, and accept others just like Jesus loves, forgives, and accepts us? Why happens when we try to express these qualities before we've experienced them?

5. What are some specific ways you can reach out to love the un-lovely and speak works of affirmation to people around you?

6. What is one act of courageous kindness you can show today?

7. If you and the believers around you were truly unified by the blood of Jesus breaking down dividing walls and building bridg-es of love, what would it look like? Is that attractive to you? Why or why not?

8

Wonder and Worship

" You were made by God and for God, and until you understand that, life will never make sense."

—**Rick Warren**

I chuckle when I think of Paul penning his connection between our grasp of the physical world and the Creator. Even without the technology we enjoy, he clearly understood the wonders of God's creation. He wrote, "For since the creation of the world God's invisible qualities—his eternal power and divine nature—have been clearly seen, being understood from what has been made, so that men are without excuse" (Romans 1:20). Paul didn't have a telescope to look at far away galaxies, and he didn't have a microscope to see the incredible intricacies of how the body works. He didn't understand the way cells generate energy, and he didn't have any idea that each type of cell in the bloodstream has a unique and crucial function. If he could walk with me for a few hours on my rounds, he would have marveled even more at God's creation.

Never Forget

Common grace and special grace. The wonder of creation and the glory of the cross. The more we understand the precision, intricacy, and beauty of the way our bodies use blood to nourish, protect, and heal, we'll marvel that God is the master architect of the vast, unimaginably expansive universe and the smallest subatomic particles. And when we look at the cross, we gaze into the heart of God. What kind of love is this, that God would become a man and die for sinful, rebellious, apathetic creatures like you and me?

In a beautiful display of symmetry, God's universe's dimension is 10^{27} meters in size, and the dimensions of the smallest subatomic particles now known are 10^{-26} meters. We fall exactly in the middle at 10^0 (which is 1, not 0). In the creation, we find immensity and minutia in perfect balance, and it fascinates us. Gerhard Staguhn comments, "He who gazes at the stars unavoidably starts thinking."[31] In the world of hematology, every time I look into a microscope, the sight of intricately crafted molecules and amazingly complex systems proclaims the glory of God to me. Even without this knowledge, Paul understood perfectly well that God inserted into creation a revelation of himself. If we'll look carefully at nature and notice its design, we'll get a glimpse of God's character and power.

I believe that scientists—from astronomers to microbiologists—have an advantage in noticing God's grand design because they study it every day. In the field of hematology, advances over the centuries have given us an ever-increasing grasp of the wonders in our blood. From ancient times, people instinctively understood that "life is in the blood." When an animal bled to death, they immediately

31 Quoted by Shirley Jones in *The Mind of God & Other Musings*, (San Rafael, CA: New World Library, 1994), p. 12.

grasped the fact that their own blood was essential to life. They also soon understood the connection between blood and health. From ancient Egypt until the 19th century, bloodletting was a common practice. Doctors thought poisons in the blood could be eliminated if the patient bled enough. The 17th century brought major advances in hematology. After van Leeuwenhoek saw different types of cells through a microscope, only a few years later, J. C. Major gave the first intravenous injection to a person, and very soon, the first transfusion was accomplished. A century later, William Hewson identified leukocytes and the clotting factor in blood. His advances won him the title: "the father of hematology." By the beginning of the 20th century, Dr. Maxwell M. Wintrobe, author of *Wintrobe's Clinical Hematology*, had enough data to set standards about the number of particular cells in a healthy person's bloodstream, paving the way for accurate diagnoses. In recent years, discoveries and treatments have increased geometrically. Today, we are discovering new insights about the way blood functions, and we are finding new ways to treat diseases related to blood. Tests on the properties of a person's blood enable doctors to detect the health or pathology of every other part of the body—thyroid, heart, lungs, kidney, liver, prostate, and so on. The human genome project, the mapping of DNA, primarily uses blood to detect the structure and order of genes, and in recent years, it has proven invaluable in detecting the real nature of diseases and disorders.

Transfusions of blood are one of the most common medical procedures today, but they are only a stopgap measure because they don't permanently solve the underlying problem for the patient. In recent years, bone marrow transplants have taken enormous strides and revolutionized the treatment of numerous diseases. We're able to identify the pluripotential stem cells and use them to address a wide range of medical problems. These cells exist not only in embryos, but also in the mature elements of a person's bloodstream. Doctors can use them to bring life and health to gravely ill patients who would have had little hope only a few years ago. The ability to use blood from all over the world is possible today because of air travel. Some physicians prefer to use blood for transfusions from particular parts of the world because certain populations have particular antibodies. But we've also learned that all blood, no matter where it originates, has amazing abilities to nourish, protect, and heal. An accident victim in the ER or a soldier on the battlefield doesn't care where the liter of blood came from. He's just thankful for its amazing properties. In every part of the hospital, medicine is advancing in phenomenal ways. I can't take Paul with me on my rounds, but I hope this book has provided you at least a peek at the wonder of God's creation, especially regarding our blood.

Paul's statement to the Roman believers means that if someone never goes to a church and never hears the gospel message, the wonder of creation is enough to convince him that there must be a Creator. One person commented, "When I realized how beautiful the world is, and I also realized how rich my life has become because of the wonders of nature—its beauty, the food I eat, family, friends, and every other physical blessing—I looked around for Someone to thank." I think Paul would smile at this comment. All of creation speaks loudly of the majesty, kindness, and glory of God, and when we look at some of the odd animals he created, we know he has a sense of humor, too.

From Genesis to Revelation

In his book, *The Chemistry of the Blood,* Dr. M. R. DeHaan observed, "The Bible is a book of blood and a bloody book. When we are accused of preaching a gospel of blood, we proudly plead guilty of the charge, for the only thing that gives life to our teaching and power to the Word of God is the fact that it is the blood, which is the very life and power of the gospel."[32] As we've seen, the first murder was described as "the shedding of blood," the old covenant of the sacrificial system promised that blood was powerful to forgive sins, and it gave strict instructions about how to handle blood. All the Old Testament directives, though, pointed to the new covenant instituted by the shedding of the blood of the perfect Lamb of God, Jesus Christ. After his death and resurrection, we might think that all this talk about death and blood would be finished, but it's not. Even in the New Heaven and New Earth, Jesus is still identified as the Lamb of God. Passover and the Lord's Table both invite us to remember the sacrificial death, the broken body and shed blood, that frees us from sin, and throughout eternity, we'll continue to reflect on the power of the Lamb's blood. Before God's throne in Revelation, the throng of believers will sing:

"You are worthy to take the scroll
*   and to open its seals,*
because you were slain,
*   and with your blood you purchased men for God*
*   from every tribe and language and people and nation.*
You have made them to be a kingdom and priests to serve our God,
*   and they will reign on the earth" (Revelation 5:9-10).*

But they aren't finished. The angels want to join the choir. In a loud voice, they all sing:

---

32 M. R. DeHaan, M. D., The Chemistry of the Blood, (Zondervan, Grand Rapids, Michigan, 1943), p. 13.

"Worthy is the Lamb, who was slain,

to receive power and wealth and wisdom and strength

and honor and glory and praise!" (Revelation 5:12)

In a paradoxical statement about the laundry in heaven, John tells us that those who have remained faithful to God and have arrived in glory "have washed their robes and made them white in the blood of the Lamb" (Revelation 7:14). The testimony of those courageous people wasn't that they were able to remain true to God on their own. They found a power source that transcended their own strength. A voice from heaven affirmed them:

"They overcame [Satan]

by the blood of the Lamb

and by the word of their testimony;

they did not love their lives so much

as to shrink from death" (Revelation 12:11).

William Cowper was often haunted by guilt, but he found peace in thinking about Christ's payment for him. He wrote some of the most beautiful and powerful hymns the church has ever known. One of them, "There is a Fountain Filled with Blood," sounds like a song that the elders, saints, and angels will sing in glory:

"There is a fountain filled with blood

drawn from Emmanuel's veins;

and sinners plunged beneath that flood

lose all their guilty stains.

Lose all their guilty stains,

lose all their guilty stains;

and sinners plunged beneath that flood

lose all their guilty stains.

E'er since, by faith, I saw the stream

thy flowing wounds supply,

redeeming love has been my theme,

and shall be till I die.

And shall be till I die,

and shall be till I die;

redeeming love has been my theme,

and shall be till I die.

Then in a nobler, sweeter song,

I'll sing thy power to save,

when this poor lisping, stammering tongue

lies silent in the grave.

Lies silent in the grave,

lies silent in the grave;

when this poor lisping, stammering tongue

lies silent in the grave."[33]

---

33 "There is a Fountain Filled with Blood," lyrics by William Cowper,
1731-1800.

Beautiful Words

The cross of Christ addresses the most profound problems facing mankind. Ultimately, our most pressing difficulties aren't our different political views or environmental problems. Those are problems we need to address, but they are secondary. The primary conundrum of the human race is the darkness in our hearts caused by sin. We may be able to manage many other problems in our lives and our society by shrewd maneuvers, but sin and spiritual death can only be addressed by a single remedy: the death of Christ. We struggle with all kinds of insecurities, but we find comfort and strength in the cross. It's the ultimate display of God's love and his good intentions for us.

The Bible uses several words to describe the impact of Christ's death in our lives. Because of his blood, we have been justified by God. *Justification* is a forensic term. We were guilty in the court of God, but Jesus paid the penalty we owed. Paul wrote, "All have sinned and fall short of the glory of God, and are justified freely by his grace through the redemption that came by Christ Jesus" (Romans 3:23-24). We don't have to be haunted by guilt and past failures. We're forgiven! Later in his letter to the Romans, Paul explained the implications: "Therefore, there is now no condemnation for those who are in Christ Jesus, because through Christ Jesus the law of the Spirit of life set me free from the law of sin and death. For what the law was powerless to do in that it was weakened by the sinful nature, God did by sending his own Son in the likeness of sinful man to be a sin offering" (Romans 8:1-3). Some of us go to church for years but still secretly wonder if we've done enough to earn entry into heaven. Surely, we fear, if God knew what we've done, he'd reject us. The truth of justification is that God knows exactly what we've done. He doesn't excuse our sin in the least. Instead, he sent Jesus to be our substitute and pay the price we could never pay. We're free!

But what good is freedom if we're alone? A second beautiful, biblical word is *reconciliation*. Before we trusted Christ, we were enemies of God—not respectable adversaries but despicable ones. However, God didn't leave us as forgiven orphans (which would have been far better than condemned sinners!). He accepted us as his own children. But that's not all. Jesus told his disciples, "I no longer call you servants, because a servant does not know his master's business. Instead, I have called you friends, for everything that I learned from my Father I have made known to you" (John 15:15). So, we have the Father for our dad and Jesus as our brother and friend. When we feel hopeless and alone, rejected by family and friends, we can be assured that the God of the universe delights in calling us his own.

When we are discouraged, anxious, angry, or when we experience any other painful emotion, we can remember these beautiful words that tell about the way the cross changes everything for us. Like the children of Israel leaving slavery in Egypt, the Passover Lamb has freed us from the slavery of sin. And like the disciples who gazed into the face of the resurrected Jesus and realized all his claims were really true, we can be confident that we belong to him. Nothing can shake these fundamental, rock-solid truths about our relationship with God.

The Necessity of Doubt

It's not wrong to ask hard questions—about the science of nature or the theology of God. In medicine, I'd wonder about the competence of any physician who wasn't inherently inquisitive. We're always learning more and finding ways to apply the truths we've learned. The spiritual world is no different. We learn and grow by thinking, asking, considering, and wondering.

We arrive at the point of assurance along the pathway of questions and doubts. Some church leaders are afraid of people asking hard questions, but Jesus welcomed honest discussion. When John the Baptist sent a messenger with a question about whether Jesus was really the One, Jesus replied, "Tell him the facts about what you've seen." We give Thomas a hard time for doubting the resurrection, but Jesus didn't condemn him. He showed his old friend the nail prints in his hands and invited him to believe. In his excellent book, *The Reason for God,* pastor Tim Keller says that honest wrestling with doubts is like white cells producing antibodies to protect against future diseases. He writes, "A faith without some doubts is like a human body without any antibodies in it. People who blithely go through life too busy or indifferent to ask hard questions about why they believe as they do will find themselves defenseless against either the experience of tragedy or the probing questions of a smart skeptic. A person's faith can collapse almost overnight if she has failed over the years to listen patiently to her own doubts, which should only be discarded after long reflection."[34]

Don't be afraid to ask questions about cosmology, physiology, psychology, theology, or any other subject. If people try to tell you that you "just need to believe," find someone who is willing to talk more deeply about the issues you've raised. In the church today, some patient, reflective people value rich dialogue about important topics, and they don't settle for simplistic answers to complex problems. A few parts of the church, however, react defensively to any question

---

34 Timothy Keller, *The Reason for God,* (Riverhead Books, New York, 2008), p. xvii.

they can't answer easily. We need to honor people who think deeply, not only the learned professors and theologians, but also the people in pews who are searching for truth.

All In or All Out

Sooner or later, we have enough answers to be able to determine whether God is trustworthy or not. We'll never have all our questions answered, and indeed, we may have even more as we grow closer to God. But at some point, we come to a conclusion about him, and the focal point of our decision is the death of Jesus. People who "play at church" don't understand that the cross isn't just the pivotal point of history; it's also the turning point of destiny for every human being. When Jesus walked the earth, people either adored him or despised him. They understood that he demanded a dramatic response to the most colossal offer the world has ever known. Nothing else will do. In his letter to the church at Laodicea, Jesus told them bluntly, "I know your deeds, that you are neither cold nor hot. I wish you were either one or the other! So, because you are lukewarm—neither hot nor cold—I am about to spit you out of my mouth" (Revelation 3:15-16). Cold food is delicious, and so is hot food. But lukewarm food is distasteful. We have more moral integrity by looking at Jesus and walking away than by treating him like a "good idea" or a "good leader." In *Mere Christianity*, C. S. Lewis famously commented, "I am trying here to prevent anyone saying the really foolish thing that people often say about Him: 'I'm ready to accept Jesus as a great moral teacher, but I don't accept His claim to be God.' That is the one thing we must not say. A man who was merely a man and said the sort of things Jesus said would not be a great moral teacher. He would either be a lunatic—on the level with the man who says he is a poached egg—or else he would be the Devil of Hell. You must make your choice. Either this man was, and is, the Son of God: or else a madman or something worse. You can shut Him up for a fool, you can spit at Him and kill Him as a demon; or you can fall at His feet and call Him Lord and God. But let us not come with any patronizing nonsense about His being a great human teacher. He has not left that open to us. He did not intend to."[35]

Love Jesus or hate him, but don't patronize him. I'm afraid that the vast majority of people in our churches each Sunday are patronizing Jesus by showing up but lacking passion for him. They don't hate him, but they only tolerate him. The message of the cross hasn't penetrated their hearts and transformed them. A friend told me that in a Bible study, the leader asked, "Why do we so quickly and easily drift back to thinking that following rules will earn us points with God?" A member of the group immediately answered, "Because we demand to be in control of our destinies." Following Jesus is both thrilling and threatening, but it's never boring. When the truth of his sacrifice for us reaches the center of our hearts, we realize that there was nothing we could do—nothing—to merit God's love and eternal life. It's entirely a free gift. But when we say yes to Christ, we give him the title to our lives. He created us and bought us. He owns us. We belong to him, and he'll take us on the adventure of our lives. True adventures always include a measure of risk, and this one is no different. We give up our demand to control our lives, and we trust God to lead us where he wants us to go and use us to accomplish his purposes. This kind of trust is the antithesis of human nature, and we have to fight the good fight every day to lay down our selfish desires and pick up our crosses as we follow Christ. Is he worthy of our affection and loyalty? That's a question all of us have to ask and answer many times in our lives.

35 C. S. Lewis, *Mere Christianity*, (Harper, San Francisco, 2001), pp. 40-41.

Amazed

The study of human blood and the blood of Jesus tells us volumes about the greatness and love of God. Both of these studies show us that God is intimately involved in meeting our deepest needs, both physically and spiritually. When we explore these two fascinating topics, our hearts are humbled by his grace and amazed by his affection. They shout that we must mean a lot to God!

Blood, ours and Christ's, is precious to God. Peter wrote, "For you know that it was not with perishable things such as silver or gold that you were redeemed from the empty way of life handed down to you from your forefathers, but with the precious blood of Christ, a lamb without blemish or defect. He was chosen before the creation of the world, but was revealed in these last times for your sake. Through him you believe in God, who raised him from the dead and glorified him, and so your faith and hope are in God" (1 Peter 1:18-21). The saints of the Old Testament could only imagine what the final sacrifice would look like. We can look back at the historical events: the life, death, and resurrection of Jesus, and marvel at his love for us.

As we close our study, let me offer a few suggestions to keep this truth from evaporating from our hearts.

When you read the Bible, look for the blood.

A friend of mine told me that after he studied the death of Christ, he began looking for references to blood and its synonyms— sacrifice, death, redemption, justification, atonement, etc.—in the New Testament letters. He said, "It's everywhere! I knew that it's the central element of his gospel, and now I realize it's the driving force of our motivation to live for Christ. It shapes our ethics and promises eternal life." When you read the Bible with this set of lenses, you'll see the blood on virtually every page.

When you take communion, take time to remember.

We sometimes treat the Lord's Table as an afterthought, and we just go through the motions. Instead, we can stop, think, and reflect on the past—the death of Christ has fully paid for all our sins and rescued us from hell; the present—his sacrifice assures us of God's never-ending love and motivates us to honor him in every way; and the future—someday, we'll dine at another meal, the Marriage Supper of the Lamb, in the New Heaven and New Earth. The Eucharist is just a taste of what's to come.

Give blood.

When we give a pint of blood or donate bone marrow for a transplant, we're giving the gift of life. Without it, people die. Depending on which procedure you choose, you may spend a few minutes or a couple of hours, but you may be giving someone a chance at life, and perhaps another opportunity to hear the gospel.

Live with joy and passion.

Let the wonderful love of God sink into your soul. Sing the hymns that remind you of God's grace poured out at the cross, and then walk out the door and love people the way God demonstrated his unconditional love for you, forgive the way he's forgiven you, and accept even the annoying people because God had enough grace to accept you.

Someone said that a lot of people around us aren't interested in Christ because they see us as hypocrites. Our walk doesn't match our talk. I know of no better medicine for this dread disease than the blood of Jesus. The most horrible means of execution has become a source of life and hope. When we look into his eyes on the cross, our defenses, pretensions, and phoniness melt away. We can be completely honest about our sins because we know we're completely loved. And when we are convinced that the grace of God reaches us, we can't wait to tell people the greatest news the world will ever hear.

Charles Wesley wrote one of his most beautiful hymns about the sacrifice of Christ. I want to close with his insights and passion about the death of our Savior.

"And can it be that I should gain

An interest in the Savior's blood?

Died He for me, who caused His pain—

For me, who Him to death pursued?

Amazing love! How can it be,

That Thou, my God, shouldst die for me?

Amazing love! How can it be,

That Thou, my God, shouldst die for me?

Long my imprisoned spirit lay,

Fast bound in sin and nature's night;

Thine eye diffused a quickening ray—

I woke, the dungeon flamed with light;

My chains fell off, my heart was free,

I rose, went forth, and followed Thee.

My chains fell off, my heart was free,

I rose, went forth, and followed Thee.

No condemnation now I dread;

Jesus, and all in Him, is mine;

Alive in Him, my living Head,

And clothed in righteousness divine,

Bold I approach th'eternal throne,

And claim the crown, through Christ my own.

Bold I approach th'eternal throne,

And claim the crown, through Christ my own.[36]

Think about it...

1. How do a better understanding of the nature of human blood
    and the sacrifice of Jesus inspire us to worship God more
    passionately?

---

36 "And Can It Be That I Should Gain?" lyrics by Charles Wesley, 1738.

2. What are some signs someone is struggling with insecurity? How do the two concepts of justification and reconciliation help resolve this pain and provide assurance?

3. Do you feel comfortable asking hard questions about God? What are some questions you've wanted to ask but were afraid to voice?

4. Which of the practical applications in this chapter (look for the blood when you read the Bible, think more deeply when you take communion, become a blood donor, and live it out) do you need to focus on today?

5. Which of the hymns in this book is most meaningful to you? How has God used it to touch your heart?

6. How will you think of blood—yours and Christ's—differently now that you've completed this study?

How to Use This Book
in Classes and Groups

This book is designed for individual study, small groups, and classes. The best way to absorb and apply these principles is for each person to individually study and answer the questions at the end of each chapter, then to discuss them in either a class or a group environment.

Each chapter's questions are designed to promote reflection, application, and discussion. Order enough copies of the book for everyone to have a copy. For couples, encourage both to have their own book so they can record their individual reflections.

A recommended schedule for a small group might be:

Week 1: Introduction to the material. The group leader can tell his own story, share his hopes for the group, and provide books for each person. Encourage people to read the assigned chapter each week and answer the questions.

Weeks 2–9: Each week, introduce the topic for the week and share a story of how God has used the principles in your life. In small groups, lead people through a discussion of the questions at the end of the chapters. In classes, teach the principles in each chapter, use personal illustrations, and invite discussion.

Personalize Each Lesson

Don't feel pressured to cover every question in your group discussions. Pick out three or four that had the biggest impact on you, and focus on those, or ask people in the group to share their responses to the questions that meant the most to them that week.

Make sure you personalize the principles and applications. At least once in each group meeting, add your own story to illustrate a particular point.

Make the Scriptures come alive. Far too often, we read the Bible like it's a phone book, with little or no emotion. Paint a vivid picture for people. Provide insights about the context of people's encounters with God, and help people in your class or group sense the emotions of specific people in each scene.

Focus on Application

The questions at the end of each chapter and your encouragement to be authentic will help your group take big steps to apply the principles they're learning. Share how you are applying the principles in particular chapters each week, and encourage them to take steps of growth, too.

Three Types of Questions

If you have led groups for a few years, you already understand the importance of using open questions to stimulate discussion. Three types of questions are *limiting, leading,* and *open.* Many of the questions at the end of each day's lessons are open questions.

- *Limiting questions* focus on an obvious answer, such as, "What does Jesus call himself in John 10:11?" These don't stimulate reflection or discussion. If you want to use questions like this, follow them with thought-provoking open questions.

- *Leading questions* sometimes require the listener to guess what the leader has in mind, such as, "Why did Jesus use the metaphor of a shepherd in John 10?" (He was probably alluding to a passage in Ezekiel, but most people wouldn't know that.)

The teacher who asks a leading question has a definite answer in mind. Instead of asking this question, he should teach the point and perhaps ask an open question about the point he has made.

• *Open questions* usually don't have right or wrong answers. They stimulate thinking, and they are far less threatening because the person answering doesn't risk ridicule for being wrong. These questions often begin with "Why do you think...?" or "What are some reasons that...?" or "How would you have felt in that situation?"

Preparation

As you prepare to teach this material in a group or class, consider these steps:

1. Carefully and thoughtfully read the book. Make notes, highlight key sections, quotes, or stories, and complete the reflection sections at the end of each day's chapter. This will familiarize you with the entire scope of the content.

2. As you prepare for each week's class or group, read the corresponding chapters again and make additional notes.

3. Tailor the amount of content to the time allotted. You won't have time to cover all the questions, so pick the ones that are most pertinent.

4. Add your own stories to personalize the message and add impact.

5. Before and during your preparation, ask God to give you wisdom, clarity, and power. Trust Him to use your group to change people's lives.

6. Most people will get far more out of the group if they read the chapters and complete the reflection each week. Order books before the group or class begins or after the first week.

About the Author

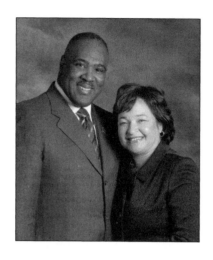

Bishop Smith was born and raised on the south side of Chicago alongside two sisters and three brothers, by his parents Shirley and Albert Smith. After the passing of Bishop Smith's mother (he was ten years old), his grandmother, Alberta Pryor, became the children's nurturing influence. She not only helped meet the needs of the children naturally, but also trained them spiritually.

His academic career includes:

- Bachelor of Science Degree (with honors) Chicago State University (1971)
- M.D., University of Illinois Medical Center (1975)
- Completion of Pediatric Residency, University of Illinois Hospital (1978)
- Completion of Clinical Fellowship in Pediatric Hematology/ Oncology at Children's Memorial Hospital/Northwestern University (1980)

On March 28, 1980, following the death of the former pastor, Bishop John S. Holly, Bishop Smith was elected pastor of Apostolic Faith Church. Under his leadership, the congregation has grown

202

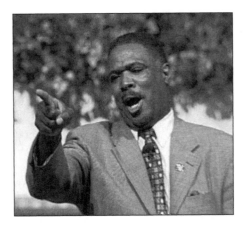

from under 200 members to over 3,000 people who call Apostolic Faith Church their home.

Bishop Smith's vision is uncompromisingly clear with one central principle —To build and develop the Kingdom of God by empowering God's people, to reach the fullest extent of their God-given potential in every area of their life. (John 10:10)

In 1997, he was elevated to the office of Bishop, and in August of 2004, Bishop Smith was elevated to the office of Presiding Bishop of the Pentecostal Assemblies of the World, Inc. (P.A.W. Inc.). The P.A.W. Inc. has over 1.5 million members worldwide, including Africa, Asia, Europe, Australia, and New Zealand.

Bishop Smith's belief in God and the power of salvation and healing extends to his medical profession as a concerned and committed pediatric hematologist-oncologist for critically ill children. He served for over 15 years as the director of the Comprehensive Sickle Cell/Thalassemia Program at Children's Memorial Hospital and is Assistant Professor of Pediatrics at Northwestern Medical School, Feinberg School of Medicine. He has been a clinical hematologist for thirty years.

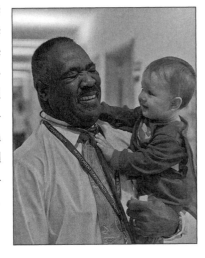

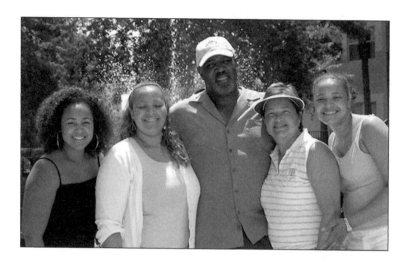

Some people believe that God and science don't mix and that faith and medicine are worlds apart. Accepting no conflict between the two worldviews, Dr. Smith believes, in fact, that ministering and medicine help him to be more effective at both. "They mix perfectly. God is the source of all knowledge," says Bishop Smith.

The principles of the Bible unlock ways of helping, healing, supporting and developing people, and impacting lives in a positive way. Combining the knowledge of both worlds blesses those he is called to serve and brings great "Glory to God." Through prayers and faith in God as a healer, Dr. Smith has seen God's healing power reverse the course of illness in the lives of his patients.

Bishop Smith has been happily married to Susan Davenport Smith since 1976. They met at the University of Illinois where Susan graduated with a B.S. in Pharmacy. They have three beautiful daughters: Lauren Elrod, Rachel Smith, and Emily Green, along with their sons-in-law, Brian Elrod, Patrick Green, and Courtney Horton, and one beautiful granddaughter, Lillian Grace Elrod, who was born January 26, 2010.

Photo Credits

To Order More Copies of This Book

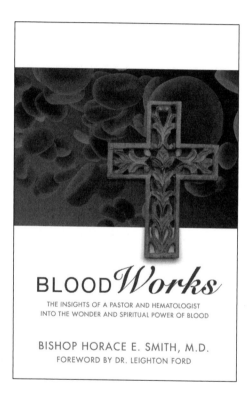

For order and discount information, go to www.afcchicago.org